Communication Skills
In Surgery

Alexander Logan MBChB MSc MR

Parjit S Dhillon MBChB MSc MRCS

© 2016 MD+ Publishing

www.mrcspartbquestions.com

Published by: MD+ Publishing

Cover Design: Alexander Logan

ISBN-10: 0993113869

ISBN-13: 978-0993113864

Printed in the United Kingdom

CONTENTS

Contributors

Preface

Chapter 1: The Basics

Chapter 2: Communication Scenarios

Chapter 3: History Taking Scenarios

Contributors

Liam Linney MBChB, BSc (Hons), MRCS
CT2 Plastic Surgery
Yorkshire and the Humber Deanery

Miss Carla Hope BMBS BMedSci MRCS
CT2 General Surgery
East Midlands Deanery

Mr Kwok-Leung Cheung
Clinical Associate Professor,
Honorary Consultant Breast Surgeon
East Midlands Deanery

David Eldred-Evans BA MA MBBS MRCS
CT2 Urology
London Deanery

Richard Goodall BSc
Fifth Year Medical Student, University of Bristol

Charlie Coughlan BA
Fifth Year Medical Student, University of Oxford

Harry Musson
Fourth Year Medical Student, Newcastle University

Alex Wilkins MBBS, B Med Sci, MRCS
Research Fellow
Hull and East Yorkshire Hospitals NHS trust

Miss Alex Murray BSc, MBChB, MRCS
CT1 Plastics
East Midlands (North) Deanery

Daniel Thurston, BSc MBBS
CT1 Trauma & Orthopaedics
East Midlands Deanery

Melanie Paul MBChB BMedSci MRCS
CT2 General Surgery
East Midlands (South) Deanery

Langhit Kurar MBChB
CT1 Orthopaedics
Kent Surrey Sussex Deanery

Aimee Rowe BSc BMBS
CT2 ENT
East Midlands North Deanery

Sarah Dawes MBChB MRCSEd(ENT)
CT1 ENT
East Midlands Deanery

Virginia Summerour BMBS MRCSEd
CT2 General Surgery
West Midlands Deanery

1 THE BASICS

THE BASICS

1.1 Introduction to Communication Skills

Communication skills stations at the MRCS examination are often thought of as the most challenging to prepare for. While most other stations require candidates to recall facts or learn examination or practical skills many candidates feel that their existing communication skills will suffice to pass communication skills scenarios and tend not to formally prepare making these some of the most challenging sections of the OSCE.

The purpose of this book is to dispel the belief that communication stations cannot be prepared for and to give you the frameworks, insights and practice scenarios to allow you to prepare alone or in small groups ahead of the MRCS Part B examination.

Getting Started

Knowing where to begin with communication skills preparation can seem daunting. Fortunately there are a limited number of potential scenarios that are likely to be assessed. Remember that these scenarios may appear in a number of contexts for example breaking bad news might involve explaining a new diagnosis of cancer to a patient or might involve explaining a patient's deterioration to a relative. Scenarios might also feature elements of more than one communication scenario type and all will require you to possess some clinical information and communicate clinical concepts in a way that can be understood by patients from non-medical backgrounds.

Types of Communication Scenario	Common History Taking Scenarios
• Breaking bad news • Discussing DNAR • Explaining a diagnosis/treatment • Obtaining consent • Dealing with an angry relative • Apologising for a mistake • Talking about clinical management • Negotiating with a difficult colleague • Supporting a struggling colleague • Cessation of smoking or alcohol	• Back pain • Dysphagia • Change in bowel habit • Osteoarthritis of hip/knee • Ischaemic limb pain • Difficulty passing urine • Anxiety

How To Improve Your Communication Skills

By using this book you are well on your way to improving your communication skills and ensuring you score highly at the assessed stations. While you will likely learn much from reading through each of the surgical communication scenarios we highly recommend practising with friends and colleagues who can use the scenarios included in the book as a script to help simulate real communication scenarios.

It is also advisable to read through your communication skills notes from medical school for further insight. Below some successful candidates who scored highly at the communication skills stations have shared their top tips:

> ✏️ **Comm Skills Tip: Tips From Candidates**
>
> - Read the scenario carefully
> - Give a confident, positive introduction to all
> - Be empathetic, don't allocate blame, remain calm and behave as you would in work
> - Actors may not be representative of the scenario (might be older/younger than patient brief)
> - You don't have long so try to finish in time
> - Provide structure: introduce, open question, listen, empathise, concerns, expectations, summarise and close
> - Stay calm and try not to become frustrated with the actor
> - Try not to argue with the actor
> - Make the actor do the work using open questions

Handling The Actors

The major limitation of any assessed communication skills examination is the use of actors rather than real patients. While the use of actors has the advantage of creating set scenarios that may be assessed, the overall interaction is false and some candidates find it difficult to take the actors seriously and act as they would do in work with real patients. Indeed the entire communication skills assessment is as much about you putting on a show for the examiners as it is about the actors themselves. Try to make yourself believe that they are a real patient and build rapport with them throughout the scenario.

> ✏️ **Comm Skills Tip: Handling The Actors**
>
> - Get them on your side
> - Greet them at the start
> - Remain calm
> - Be unreactive
> - Take it seriously
> - Make them do the work

1.2   What Are Communication Skills?

Communication skills can be divided into three key concepts: non-verbal communication techniques (body language), verbal communication techniques and verbal content. In essence these can be thought of as your body language, your manner of speech and the content of your speech.

Non-Verbal Communication Skills (Body Language)

Body language is extremely important and plays a pivotal role in effective communication. It can be difficult to know how to sit, who to look at or what to do with your arms during an assessed communication scenario. While much of this is common sense and you will, hopefully, have developed and built upon your awareness of non-verbal communication skills taught at medical school it is important to cover the basics so that under pressure you are able to maintain appropriate body language and score highly during assessment.

Sitting

A number of studies have identified the position of sitting slightly forward feet planted on the ground with hands crossed or fingers locked and forearms resting on your thighs as being the optimum position for demonstrating engagement when communicating with another individual. This position makes you look calm and ready and is in between leaning in too far and slouching back in your chair. This position can be maintained for the majority of the scenario and allows you to sit back slightly between responses from the actor and at the end of the station.

Smile

While you will be nervous, a soft smile will help to put the actor at ease and will help you to build rapport during the station.

Eye Contact

Ensure that you make eye contact with the actor from the start. If you find holding eye contact difficult practice focusing on peoples' eyebrows when you talk to them (the eye of the other person cannot discriminate whether you are looking at their eye or eyebrow due to proximity). When listening to the actor nod to show understanding and when giving your information make sure you maintain eye contact with all the actor and do not look up or down when trying to recall information.

Hands

From the initial handshake to using hand gestures to enforce or explain points your hands can help to demonstrate confidence and conviction if used correctly. Upon entering the room respond to handshakes if offered and look the actor in the eyes. Keep your hands on your knees or lap when listening to the conversation and raise them when explaining a point.

Active Listening

When being asked questions or listening to the actor sit attentively. Movements such as tilting your head or nodding in understanding demonstrate active listening and will make you appear more engaging to the actor. Try to avoid using too many 'verbal fillers' such as 'Mmmm' or 'Uh-huh'. While these might demonstrate that you are listening they can also interrupt the actor.

Mirroring

This is an advanced body language technique in which you subtly copy or 'mirror' the body language of the actor. Mirroring can establish rapport with the individual who is being mirrored, as the similarities in nonverbal gestures allow the individual to feel more connected with the person exhibiting the mirrored behavior.

Verbal Communication Skills

Once you have mastered body language it is time to analyse how you deliver your responses. An excellent explanation delivered in a quiet, stuttering manner will score less than one delivered in a confident and assured manner.

Vocal Clarity

Project your voice in a conversational manner, sit upright and speak clearly. You will be nervous initially and may hear your voice waiver. This is entirely normal and you will settle in to things after you begin speaking. Speak loudly and clearly enough to be heard by both actor and assessor.

Length of Response

Stopping yourself from talking when nervous can be extremely difficult, however, when explaining a diagnosis or answering a question try to deliver the information in manageable, chunks to facilitate understanding. Most structured points can be given within 2-3 minutes leaving time for further questions.

Speed

Some people talk quickly others talk slowly. When you are under pressure this will likely be exaggerated. Try to find a balance and don't be afraid to pause or allow for silence.

Vocal Tonality

Changing your inflection and emphasising words prevents listeners from getting bored. Think about how quickly you lose interest when speaking to someone talking about something in a monotonous, single tone voice and then think about someone who changes their tone and emphasises words. This will help you to build rapport with the actor and keep the assessor engaged.

Enthusiasm

Following on from tonality and word emphasis make sure that you are positive and enthusiastic when communicating with the actor. Smiling and tonality make up a large portion of this and the rest is about overcoming nerves and trying to put the actor at ease. Ensure, however, that your demeanor is appropriate to the topic of the scenario.

Verbal Content Skills

Now that you understand some of the more esoteric communication skill concepts it is time to focus on what you say to the patient/actor.

Connecting

Build rapport and get the actor on side. The above body language and verbal techniques such as smiling, mirroring and vocal tonality will help you persuade the actor that you are a confident, understanding individual who is there to help them. In essence you want to convey that you are there to assist the actor with their problems and concerns as best you can and can empathise with their predicament.

✎ Comm Skills Tip: How To Build Rapport

You will often hear the word rapport used in communication skills. Rapport is a relationships in which both parties have confidence in each other, mutual respect and confidence. During the consultation you are tasked with building rapport with the patient/actor. Below are some practical ways to do this in a short space of time:

• Smile
• Begin with a proper introduction
• Show respect, allow them to talk and listen when they do
• Relate: say you understand and empathise
• Acknowledge their concerns
• Agree with them
• Involve the patient/actor in decisions
• Provide help
• Provide a plan that both of you agree upon

Open Questions

Open questions allow the actor to provide you with the information that they feel is most pertinent and appropriate rather than simply answering questions you judge to be relevant. As you will read later on we recommend beginning with two open questions to ensure the actor divulges as much information as possible from the start. Try to make the actor do the work and focus on active listening techniques while they talk.

Empathy

Demonstrating that you can see things from the actor's point of view and understand their concerns is extremely important. While you may not have directly experienced their situation yourself you can at the very least appreciate the severity or importance of the problem that the patient or actor is facing. You can demonstrate empathy through your body language and non-verbal skills by nodding understandingly and through active listening and can more overtly demonstrate empathy with your content by using phrases such as 'that must have been difficult for you' or 'I am sorry that this has happened' or by reflecting back what the actor has already mentioned. Try to avoid directly saying 'I understand' since it is unlikely you have had a similar experience yourself and this can come across as patronizing.

Comm Skills Tip: How To Demonstrate Empathy

The following phrases show practical ways that you can use verbal content to demonstrate empathy in your conversation:

- "I realize how complicated it is to…"
- "This must be very difficult for you…"
- "I cannot imagine how upsetting it is to…"
- "It must be confusing when…"
- "I'm so sorry to hear that…"
- "I'm sorry that it isn't better news."
- "I'm glad you came today so that we can take care of this right away."

Reflecting

An empathetic response accurately identifies the factual content of the actor or patient's statement, as well as the nature and intensity of their feelings, concerns, or expectations. A reflection of content (symptoms or ideas) might sound like the following:
'So you were fine until this morning when you woke up with back pain, and it's been getting more severe ever since?'
'You're worried that you might have cancer and will need to have chemotherapy'
You may also mirror the patient's interests and values:
'So, if I understand correctly, what you really enjoy is going out at night with your friends and having a few drinks?'

Warning Shot

Prepare the actor for what you are about to tell them by giving them a subtle hint earlier in the exchange of what is to come. A warning shot is most useful when breaking bad news. For example rather than immediately giving a concerning diagnosis you may wish to forewarn the patient by saying 'I am sorry but it is not good news…' or by using subtly negative wording such as 'unfortunately, I have read the scan report and…'. This is most effective when coupled with an appropriate tone of voice, facial expression and general demeanor.

Sign-Posting

Sign-posting can be used to structure your side of the consultation and explain what information you will be giving and what you need to find out from the patient. By providing a structured approach the actor will be put at ease and may even follow the structure without further prompting from you. An example of sign-posting might simply be to say 'I would first like to ask you a few questions about your condition, then find out what your concerns are before we then both decide upon where we go from here'.

Handing Over

Give the actor responsibility in any management plan formulated and make sure he or she is happy with the outcome. It is highly recommended that you use open questions and make the actor do the work in the station rather than being too paternalistic in your plan. Remember you are merely there to guide the actor through the station and formulate a plan together.

Safety Netting

Forming a management plan is the end goal of any assessed communication scenario. A

THE BASICS

good plan will take into account any unexpected problems and try to reduce any uncertainty on the patient. Simply saying that you will arrange to see the patient again at a follow up appointment to ensure their symptoms have not changed is safety netting. Other safety nets might include involving multidisciplinary team members to provide support for a patient's needs, offering to discuss results with a senior colleague and then return and inform the patient of this or simply stating that the patient will be reviewed regularly in hospital.

Be Direct

Give information in a clear and direct manner. Use sign-posting and warning shots to structure and soften the information given but when actually giving the information ensure that you get to the point and there is no confusion regarding the information or its implications to the patient.

Keep It Simple

Keep things simple and avoid too much jargon especially when explaining a procedure or consenting a patient for an operation.

Silence

Occasionally the actor may go silent. This most commonly occurs if you have delivered some bad news. Do not feel as though you need to talk to fill the silence but rather allow the actor time to process the information. When they have had a little time to process the information they will likely begin to ask questions.

Summarising and Clarifying

Summarising what the actor has told you helps to ensure that you have not missed any important facts and that they are correct. Summarising also helps to improve rapport by explicitly demonstrating to the actor that you have been listening and have picked up upon the most salient points. Summarising is best done immediately prior to formulating a management plan and helps to clarify that nothing important has been missed and that the actor is happy to proceed and does not wish to offer anything further.

✎ Comm Skills Tip: Remembering The Key Principles

It can be difficult to remember all of the above principles and tricky to practically implement them in a consultation at first. When beginning try to focus on a few key principles using the S C O R E S acronym:

- **S**ilence
- **C**larifying
- **O**pen Questions
- **R**eflecting Back
- **E**mpathetic Comments
- **S**ummarising

1.3 Communication Skills Frameworks

In order to perform well at communication skills OSCE stations it is important that you have a framework that can be utilized when approaching any type of communication scenario.

In 1984 social psychologist David Pendleton wrote his PhD thesis on the analysis of the patient consultation and this was the basis for the now widely used Calgary-Cambridge model of patient consultation.

THE BASICS

The Calgary-Cambridge Model of Communication

The Calgary-Cambridge model divides the consultation into 'tasks' and provides a framework for ensuring rapport is built, appropriate information is gathered, explanations are provided and a plan is created.

The consultation is divided into:

- **Initiating the session** (rapport, reasons for consulting, establishing shared agenda).
- **Gathering information** (patient's story, open and closed questions, identifying verbal and non-verbal cues).
- **Building the relationship** (developing rapport, recording notes, accepting the patient's views/feelings and demonstrating empathy and support).
- **Explanation and planning** (giving digestible information and explanations).
- **Closing the session** (summarising and clarifying the agreed plan).

The Calgary-Cambridge framework can be used for any communication skills scenario and features the key components against which you will be assessed at surgical OSCE stations. You should see yourself as a guide moving the actor through the different stages of the framework before agreeing upon a plan together. Try and make the actor do the majority of the work by using open questions, asking for their opinion at all stages and getting them to decide upon their chosen course of action after you have provided appropriate medical information. Guide the actor and when you are required to speak (providing medical information or answering questions) keep it simple, jargon-free and on-point.

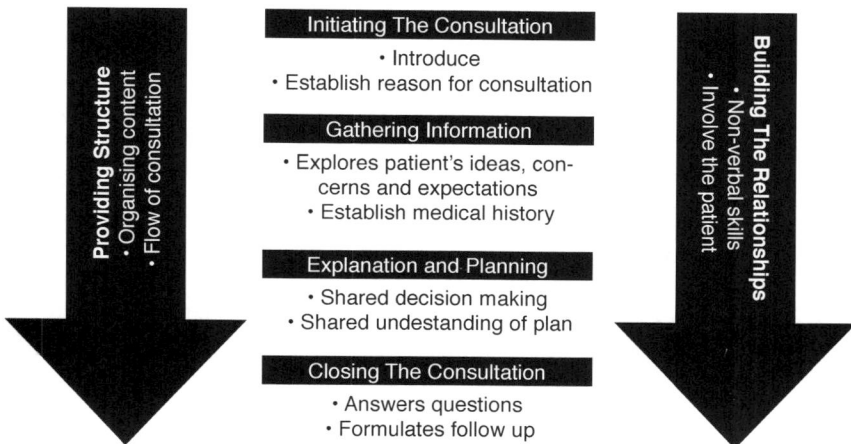

Providing Structure
- Organising content
- Flow of consultation

Initiating The Consultation
- Introduce
- Establish reason for consultation

Gathering Information
- Explores patient's ideas, concerns and expectations
- Establish medical history

Explanation and Planning
- Shared decision making
- Shared understanding of plan

Closing The Consultation
- Answers questions
- Formulates follow up

Building The Relationships
- Non-verbal skills
- Involve the patient

For the purpose of ensuring all scoring domains are covered for the OSCE we have adapted the above framework into one specifically for the short, assessed communication skills stations of an OSCE.

Introduce, open question, listen, empathise, concerns, expectations, summarise and close

Step	What You Do
1) Introduction	Say 'Hello'
2) Gather information	What's the problem? (x2 open questions)
3) Consider problem	Listen
4) Ideas, concerns and expectations	How can I help? (ICE)
5) Detail treatment or investigation	Provide appropriate information
6) Check understanding	Clarify understanding and summarise
7) Plan and close	Plan, safety net and say goodbye

Breaking Down Any Communication Scenario

The above modified Calgary-Cambridge framework can be used for both specific types of communication scenarios, such as breaking bad news, and also for history taking stations.

Knowing how to practically implement this framework as a guide while maintaining your natural flow of conversation and not coming across as too robotic may seem like a challenge. As you practise try to consider what stage of the consultation you are at and think back to previous communication scenarios you have done or conversations with patients in work and reflect on which components of the framework you already use.

We have broken down the framework into its core components and discuss each in more detail in the following section.

The Scenario

Your tasks:
- Carefully read the scenario
- Mentally note key information such as names, scan results etc.

The Introduction

Your tasks:
- Make sure you properly introduce yourself and have the correct patient
- Have as much background information as possible before starting
- Make sure the actor is happy and ready to talk (gaining consent)

Checklist
- Acknowledge everyone in the room
- When you are asked to start introduce yourself
- Shake hands, make eye contact
- State your name and role
- Clarify their name

- State what you have been tasked to do
- Check that they are happy to proceed

Gathering Information

Your tasks:
- This is the key to all of the rest of the station
- Get this right and it all flows
- Get it wrong and it all goes wrong
- Miss it out at your peril even for what appears to be an explanation station

Checklist
- Start with an open question
- What is/are the task(s) or problem(s)?
- Remember that there is usually more than one
- You need to be sure you get all of them
- You need to move on from here to the actor's perspective (ICE)

Consider the problem (listen)

Your tasks:
- Demonstrate active listening

Checklist
- Listen – let them talk
- When the actor stops let them know you have heard it all (mini summary)
- Screen for any other issues: 'anything else?'
- Before moving to closed questions explain why you are asking closed questions (sign-post)
- Ask closed questions relevant to the problems discussed
- Summarise and check all that you have found out thus far

Ideas, Concerns and Expectations (ICE)

Your tasks:
- You want to know about:
    - What they are worried or think might be going on?
    - What they already know or have been told?
    - How it is affecting their lives/ day to day functioning?
    - What they were expecting from you?
- Manage their ideas, concerns and expectations
- Work **with** the actor to make decisions

Checklist
- Pick up cues: "you mentioned…"
- Acknowledge their concerns
- Be non judgmental
- Do not make assumptions about the problem or the actor's agenda
- Make sure you understand where they are coming from
- Use empathy: 'I can see that it is difficult for you'
- Always involve the actor

Provide Information

Your tasks:
• Deliver the required information in simple, direct terms
• Facilitate understanding

Checklist
• Break down the information into simple chunks
• Signpost how many important bits there are to convey (warning shot as in breaking bad news)
• Explain one at a time (finger counting)
• Integrate it into the actor's framework
• Use hand gestures if required

Check Understanding

Your tasks:
• Summarise and clarify all that has been discussed

Checklist
• Check the actor understands and agrees
• Allow opportunity to ask questions
• Summarise and clarify
• Get the actor to add any additional information

Plan and Close

Your tasks:
• Formulate a combined plan
• Organise follow up
• Close the station

Checklist
• Safety net by making a shared plan or follow up meeting
• Explain the plan
• Agree the plan with the actor
• Check they understand the plan
• Thank the actor

What to Do If You Get Stuck

Candidates who perform poorly usually do so because they have missed out important information or have not ascertained what is important to the actor. In some scenarios actors are given briefs with information that they will not divulge unless given the appropriate opportunity to do so. An example of this might be a patient concerned about a routine operation because their relative had a bad experience in the past.

Other troublesome scenarios might be when an actor presses you for information that you just don't have such as the specifics of an operation or demanding for something to happen. In any situation where you do not have all of the facts at hand the best policy is to be honest. Say that you do not know and do not want to provide inaccurate information but that you realise that the information is important to the actor and you will endeavour to find out after the scenario and then come back and inform them.

✎ Comm Skills Tip: How To Not Get Stuck

• Get into the habit of having a structure in mind
• When things seem to be going wrong it is usually because you are not sure where the actor is coming from and so go back to gathering information
• Go back to finding out the actor's perspective using ICE

1.4 Specific Scenario Types

This book provides many different types of scenarios for you to practise. Some feature multiple communication tasks such as breaking bad news, explaining a diagnosis and more. This section briefly covers the key points to the most commonly assessed types of communication skills tasks to enable you to quickly recall the key elements unique to each.

Breaking Bad News

Breaking bad news can come in many forms: explaining a test result, explaining the death of a relative, explaining the spread of a cancer or delivering any unwanted news that you might have to tell a patient or relative.

Breaking bad news is a common communication skills scenario but can be daunting as no one wants the patient or actor to become upset. Knowing how to effectively prepare the patient and deliver the bad news is a skill. Having a framework is useful and the Cambridge-Calgary or the breaking bad news-specific **SPIKES** protocol can be employed.

SPIKES is a six-step protocol which has been shown to improve the confidence of clinicians who use it when breaking bad news to cancer patients:
• **Setting up** the interview.
• Assessing the patient's **Perception**.
• Obtaining the patient's **Invitation**, as shunning information is a valid psychological coping mechanism.
• Giving **Knowledge** and information to the patient.
• Addressing the patient's **Emotions with Empathetic** response.
• Having a **Strategy and Summarising**.

In essence you can think of this as:

Setting: Having the discussion in a quiet environment, removing your bleep and asking if they would like a nurse or family member present (often this can be skipped in the OSCE setting)

Perception: Asking what they know thus far and what they are concerned about
"Can you tell me what you have been told thus far? Is there anything that is of particular concern to you?"

Invitation: Explaining that you are there to deliver the news and also the management plan going forward
"I am here to explain the test results to you is that OK?"
Some patients might not want to know but it is important that they do so that they can make an informed decision regarding subsequent treatment.

Knowledge: Providing the patient with the bad news using a warning shot to lessen the blow:
"I'm afraid it is not good news. The test results have shown that it is a cancer."

Emotions and Empathy: Explaining that you understand it must be difficult to hear and give the patient time to process the information:
"I am sorry. I know this must be very difficult to hear. Please take a moment."

Strategy and Summarising: Explaining that there is a plan going forward:
"The results will be discussed at the oncology MDT and our cancer specialist nurse will come and speak with you. We will see what treatment is appropriate and provide you with further information after this."

Most people get stuck at 'K' when delivering the news. Ensure you use a warning shot but then deliver the news directly. If it is cancer or that someone has died say so. Trying to use 'softer' words such as lesion or tumour can add confusion to an already difficult conversation and lead to false hope.

✏️ Comm Skills Tip: Breaking Bad News Tips

- Warning shot
- Say you are sorry
- Be direct
- Silence: allow time to process
- Positive, shared plan
- Empathy: 'I realise this is difficult for you...'
- Safety net with follow up
- Say you are sorry again
- Follow up and what to do next

Angry Patient/Relative

Dealing with anger is a scary scenario to encounter in work and even more so under pressure during an OSCE. The key to dealing with anger is to realise that there is usually an underlying reason why the person is angry. Allow the individual the opportunity to vent their anger without interruption. Being angry takes quite a lot of effort and is difficult to maintain. Once the actor or patient has vented their frustration try to appreciate why they are angry. Use empathy to build rapport and apologise for any situation that has caused the anger.

The actor may have been instructed to remain angry for the whole station and the only resolution may be directing them towards the PALS service. Often angry individuals will demand things such as speaking with the consultant or wanting the name of an individual nurse or doctor. Though it can be intimidating, remember to stick to your guns, explain that these things are not possible and again point them towards PALS.

Comm Skills Tip: Dealing With Anger

- Open question
- Allow time to vent anger
- Sit patient down
- Mirror body language
- Agree with the actor/patient
- Apologise but do not allocate blame
- Establish their main concerns (what is the underlying reason they are angry?)
- Establish a plan
- Apologise again as they may not have acknowledged your first apology
- Offer PALS service

Explaining A Diagnosis Or Treatment

Explaining a diagnosis hinges on two main factors: using understandable terms and having knowledge of the diagnosis or treatment. The former can be tricky for some as doctors are used to using certain terms when talking about medical conditions. Knowledge of the condition must come from your existing knowledge base but if the patient asks you for specific information that you do not have (such as the precise risk of a complication) it is acceptable to do as you would in work and be honest stating that you do not know but that you will endeavour to find out.

Comm Skills Tip: Explaining

- Establish patient background
- Establish what the patient has been told
- Establish what they understand
- ICE
- Is there a particular reason they are concerned?
- Explain in simple terms
- Clarify understanding
- Summarise

Consent

Similar to explaining a diagnosis or treatment it is important that you have an existing knowledge base so that you can accurately explain the benefits and risks. If the station specifically states that the patient must sign the consent form make sure that you do just that and don't waste time talking about their medical history which will not score you points.

Try to structure the risks to aid recollection. An example of this might be general complications, such as infection, thrombosis etc, and procedure specific, such as dislocation in hip replacements or anastomotic leak in a Hartmann's procedure.

THE BASICS

Comm Skills Tip: Consent

- Revise key operation risks
- Hip fractures, arthroplasty, cholecystectomy and scopes in detail
- If asked a specific percentage risk that you are unsure about say so but say you will find out
- Confirm patient name and date of birth
- Find out background and existing knowledge
- If the scenario states they need to sign the form make sure they sign it

Struggling Colleague

Occasionally you may be asked to talk with a colleague as there has been a dispute or problem flagged up by another colleague or staff member. There is often an underlying issue at play ranging from problems at home to a doctor being unable to cope with the workload. Be non-judgmental and gather information sensitively before offering support and help if required. You do not need to escalate everything to a more senior colleague but rather ask the struggling individual if they think discussing the matter with their consultant or supervisor would be of benefit and allow them to make the decision themselves, respecting their autonomy.

Comm Skills Tip: Struggling Colleague

- Build rapport
- Ask how they think they are doing in work and out of work
- Ask if they have spoken with friends/colleagues
- Information gathering key is key to identify reasons behind their struggle
- Set goals
- Involve educational supervisor if appropriate

Apologising

Apologising for a mistake often incorporates elements of breaking bad news and dealing with anger. Mistakes are often unavoidable and it may simply be that the patient has developed a complication, which was previously explained during the consent process. Remember not to allocate or accept blame yourself but rather apologise for the situation the patient has found himself or herself in. An angry person may not acknowledge your apology at first so remember to repeat the apology once they have become more reasonable. Explain that all complications or errors are followed up and reassure the patient that you will endeavour to rectify their complication. The patient may still want to complain even after your apology and should be directed to the PALS service.

🖉 Comm Skills Tip: Apologising

- Find out what the actor knows
- Listen to how the mistake or problem has affected them
- Ensure you know all their concerns
- Then apologise
- Do not fall on your sword or allocate blame
- Reassure that it is being acted upon to prevent further errors
- Involve the patient/actor in the plan
- Apologise again

Negotiating

Whether the scenario requires you to convince a difficult patient to not self-discharge, to take a treatment or to request a scan from an obstructive colleague negotiating requires you to build rapport and explain why the individual should change their mind and consider your alternative.

🖉 Comm Skills Tip: Negotiating

- Build rapport
- Explain why you need their cooperation
- Explain what you need from them
- Elicit why they are being unhelpful
- If still obstructive re-iterate the need for help
- If still obstructive involve a senior

2 COMMUNICATION

2.1 Cholangiocarcinoma Results

Scenario

You are the CT2 on the ward. Mrs. Smith is a 54-year-old lady who was admitted with right upper quadrant pain, jaundice and weight loss. She has had a CT scan which has shown a likely cholangiocarcinoma. Your Consultant has asked you to explain the scan results to her.

Both you and the patient are in a quiet side room and a nurse is present with you. You have given your bleep to a colleague to avoid interruptions. You have washed your hands and introduced yourself.
Please explain the diagnosis to the patient.

How would you begin?

Open the conversation by telling the patient that you are here to discuss their scan results, so that the patient knows what to expect.

You: "Hello Mrs. Smith, my name is Dr. X and I work for Mr. Jones, your Consultant. I have come to explain your scan results to you"

Ascertain how much information the patient already knows

Encourage them to tell you what they know so far so that you can gauge their ideas, concerns and expectations. The patient may divulge a suspicion of cancer at this time.

You: "Before we go any further, could I just check with you what you know so far?"

66 **Patient:** *"Well, I've had this pain on the right side for a while, which has gotten worse and I've started to turn yellow. I've had a scan as I know you Doctors are concerned it may be something serious. Honestly, I am really worried it could be cancer."*

How would you then proceed?

Ask the patient if they would like to have a friend or relative present. Double check that the environment is right for them to receive the news and that they wish to hear it. This also serves as a first warning shot to the patient that this is bad news.

You: "Would you like me to go through the scan results and explain everything to you? Would you like to have anyone with you whilst we talk about this?"

66 **Patient:** *"My husband won't be here until later, but I can't wait any longer, please just tell me the news. Worrying about it has been the worst thing. I just want to know what's wrong."*

You: "I'm sorry but the scan results are not what we had hoped for and the appearance is of a cancer"

> ✏️ **Comm Skills Tip: Breaking Cancer Diagnosis**
>
> Deliver the news briefly with simple language. Avoid using terms like 'malignancy' or 'neoplasm'. The words 'tumour' and 'growth' can be used as a warning shot at the start of the sentence but this should always be clarified as 'cancer'.

What will you do next?

Allow the patient time to digest the information. After delivering the news give the patient some time to process it. They may look shocked, have an emotional response or you may sit in silence for a time. They may continue to speak to you in normal conversation, but bear in mind the impact this news will have had on them and keep further conversation in simple language. Remember that most of what you say subsequently will be forgotten by the patient but it is important to answer their questions honestly.

❝ **Patient:** *"Am I going to die?" [This is a dreaded question, remember to be honest but not destroy hope]*

You: "I understand this must have come as quite a shock and this is a difficult conversation to have. We will be able to offer you some treatment. This type of cancer usually requires surgery to treat it. Part of the treatment we give will focus on helping with your symptoms, such as good management of your pain."

❝ **Patient:** *"Give it to me straight Doctor, what are my odds?"*

You: "We need to know some more information before we can be certain what the prognosis is and I will need to speak to my Consultant, the Radiology Doctors and the Oncology Doctors. We will need to decide whether we are able to perform surgery to remove your tumour. If we can, the 5-year survival is between 25 and 50 percent, although this will depend on various things such as whether the cancer has spread. I don't want to overload you with information as all this will be a lot to take in but we can discuss this again in the future."

You can explain that in surgically resectable disease the 5 year survival is 25-50% however this depends on multiple variable such as nodal status, degree of local spread and choice of surgical procedure. Whilst you do not want to 'dodge the question' it is important to reiterate that there are as yet unknown variables and that the management will be a team decision. You should also gauge the patient's response, it is unlikely they will be able to retain specific information following the bad news and it is sensible to state that you can discuss this further in the future with them.

> ✏️ **Comm Skills Tip: Empathy For A Diagnosis**
>
> It is acceptable to say that you are 'sorry' for the diagnosis. Do not say that you understand what they are going through, as although this is empathetic it may not be true. It is better to say that you understand this is a difficult diagnosis to hear.

COMMUNICATION

Having delivered the news how will you proceed?

Let the patient lead the consultation. There may be a period of silence.

66 **Patient:** *"So, what's next Doctor?"*

You: "The Consultant, Mr. Jones, will need to discuss today's scan at the meeting with the Radiology Doctors and the Oncology Doctors. We can then make decisions about how best to treat the cancer. In the mean time I will call the cancer specialist nurse to come and speak with you.

We can help you manage the pain with medication and give you intravenous fluids to help you feel better. We will also do further blood tests. After the meeting the decision may be that more scans are required."

What will you ask next?

The patient may have specific questions, which you should answer sensitively and honestly, or they may have no questions.

You: "Do you have any questions?"

66 **Patient:** *"Will I definitely need surgery?"*

You: "The best way to treat these tumours is with surgery and chemotherapy, although not all tumours are operable. We will need to look carefully at all of your scans before we make decisions about surgery, but it may be an option."

66 **Patient:** *"Is it a big surgery?"*

You: "The surgery required can be complex, but we will speak to you about this once we have had the meeting"

66 **Relative:** *"Will I need chemotherapy? Will my hair fall out?"*

You: "Chemotherapy may form part of the treatment that we give. After the meeting the Oncology doctor will come and speak to you about the best kind of chemotherapy to use and will explain all of the side effects."

What would you do next?

Once the patient has asked questions and you have answered to the best of your ability it is important to check that they have sufficient support in place and clarify their understanding prior to closing the consultation.

You: "Do you have anyone you would like to call or that I can call to come in?"

66 **Patient:** *"No, it's OK. My husband will be in later"*

You: "Would you like myself and the Nurse to stay with you for a while?"

66 **Patient:** *"Actually, could the nurse stay for a while? I just don't want to be on my own."*

COMMUNICATION

You: "Is there anything else I can do for you?"

66 **Patient:** *"Please just keep me up to date with what you are planning to do. Also, would you be able to come back later to speak to my husband?"*

You: "Certainly Mrs. Smith. I will ask the nurses to let me know when your husband arrives and I will try to speak to my Consultant before this and update you. I will also check your fluid chart and drug chart to ensure you have the correct medications prescribed"

66 **Patient:** *"Thank you."*

How would you close the consultation?

It is nice to close the consultation by confirming the bad news but giving a safety net and a plan. Before leaving ensure that the patient knows how to contact you should they have further questions i.e. they can ask the ward staff to bleep you. Say that you will return later in the day to speak to them again, appreciating that they will have thought of more questions after you leave. Offer to return to speak to friends or relatives (they often have more questions than the patient!) and ensure that the ward has your contact details.

You: "I'm sorry that this was bad news and is a lot to take in. I'm going now to speak with the cancer specialist nurse and ask her to come and visit you. We will let you know as soon as we have more information about the next steps. I will come back later this afternoon to speak with you and your husband."

SUMMARY

Setting up the environment has been done for you in this scenario but, if it is not, always offer not only a chaperone but a figure that can offer support such as a Specialist Nurse. Always ensure that the environment will be free form interruptions, such as your bleep, and away from the hustle and bustle of the ward activity.

Structure the consultation. At the start it is helpful to 'fire a warning shot' so that the patient has a chance to brace for bad news. State clearly and succinctly what the bad news is and do not shy away from the word 'cancer'. After the bad news allow a period of silence to let the news sink in, ideally the patient should break this silence.
It is important never to lie to a patient, if you do not know something say that you do not know but offer to find out and arrange to get back to them with the information. Do not give false promises, do not say 'everything will be OK' as this is false reassurance. Equally never destroy hope for a patient; you will always be able to offer something even if treatment is not for longevity.

When closing the consultation you must plan follow up actions. These will always involve MDT discussion for cancer diagnoses and referral to Macmillan or Oncology Specialist Nurses should be made. Always offer to return at a later time in anticipation of questions and to speak to relatives.

😐 **Actor Brief**

Mrs. Smith is a 54-year-old accountant who has had pain in her right upper quadrant, has begun to turn yellow and has lost 3 stone over the past 6 months. She is anxious about a diagnosis of cancer as her son is a medical student and she has also looked online for causes of her symptoms. She is a quite an anxious person and wants to know the diagnosis and plan as quickly as possible.

Special Instructions: The actor should cry and go silent upon being told the diagnosis. They will then want to know specifically about the next steps.

TOP TIPS

➕ Silent periods will always feel longer than they are; try counting 1-Mississippi-2-Mississsppi-3-Mississippi in your head if you struggle with leaving silent periods.

➕ Empathy is very important in these scenarios. Remember to use open body language. Touching a patient is acceptable, for example on the shoulder, however if this does not come naturally to you this is best avoided.

➕ Honesty is the best policy, but be careful not to destroy hope. The prognosis for cholangiocarcinoma is very poor in non-resectable disease, although this does not mean that we do not give treatment. Treatment in any cancer will either be with curative or palliative intent.

2.2 | Death Of A Relative

Scenario

You are the CT2 on-call for surgery overnight. At midnight Mr. Shardlow, a 66-year-old gentleman, was admitted as an emergency with a ruptured Abdominal Aortic Aneurysm. He was rushed to theatre for surgery but unfortunately suffered cardiac arrest and died whilst on the table. Your Consultant Miss Banks is documenting the operation and has asked you to go and speak to the family.

Mr. Shardlow's wife and daughter are waiting for you in the quiet room on the Surgical Assessment Unit. A Nurse has accompanied you to see them. You have washed your hands and introduced yourself. Please explain to the family what has happened.

How would you begin?

In real life people will often be able to tell from your demeanor that it is not good news. You have already ensured that the environment is suitable to deliver this news and that a Nurse is present with you. You may not be able to start the scenario as the relatives may ask you first what has happened.

You: "Hello my name is Dr. X. I am one of the surgical doctors. Could I begin by asking what you have been told so far?"

❝ **Relative:** *"My father became very unwell with stomach pains a few hours ago and it was so bad we called an ambulance. The emergency doctors told us they thought he had a ruptured aneurysm and needed emergency surgery and then we spoke to one of your colleagues who explained that it was quite serious. We are just so worried. Has the surgery been okay?"*

You: "It is not good news I am afraid. I'm so sorry to have to tell you, your father has not survived the operation."

At this point there can be a variety of reactions; the most likely is that the family members will become upset. It may feel uncomfortable but you need to leave a silence here and allow the relative to dictate how the consultation continues.

✏ Comm Skills Tip: Handling Crying

Some people can find this situation very awkward. Consider your body language and keep your demeanor open and supportive. You need to take cues from the person you are speaking with. If physical contact feels natural it is appropriate to place a hand on their shoulder, however if this does not feel natural avoid physical contact. You can offer tissues but don't force them. Sit quietly with the family and allow them to express their grief.

Allow an appropriate period of silence before continuing the consultation.

COMMUNICATION

How would you proceed?

After a respectful period of silence, gently move the consultation on. At this point it is kind to say something reassuring, for example that the relative was not in any pain or distress. Reassure that you 'did everything you could'. You can then move on to see if there are any questions.

You: "I'm so sorry for your loss. We did all we could and he was not in any pain when he passed. I'm sure you have questions and I will answer them for you as best I can."

66 **Relative:** *"What happened?"*

You: "Your husband had suffered from a ruptured aneurysm, which is when the main blood vessel in the body balloons out over time and can then burst. This leads to severe and sudden internal bleeding. Sometimes we can catch it in time and fix it with surgery. Often we cannot."

66 **Relative:** *"Was there nothing more that you could have done? Why did you give up on him?"*

You: "As soon he arrived we took him straight to theatre for emergency surgery. We replaced the lost blood with fluids and blood transfusions. The surgical team tried to repair the burst aneurysm. We continued to give fluids, blood transfusions and drugs to help support him, but your husband's heart stopped and we were not able to restart it despite our best efforts."

66 **Relative:** *"How did this happen? He was fine yesterday, he was a healthy man. He had a scan for aneurysm last year and we were told it was small and would be monitored."*

You: "Sometimes people develop these dilations in the main blood vessel and because they do not have any symptoms we screen for them. If they are small we keep a watchful eye on them but sometimes they can get very big very quickly. If this happens they are at high risk of bursting, which is unfortunately what seems to have happened in your husband's case. The events surrounding his death will be looked into by the coroner to ensure that we did not miss anything."

66 **Relatives:** *"The coroner? Does that mean an autopsy? This is too much to take in."*

You: "I'm sorry that it is a lot of information. I'll briefly explain what referral to the coroner involves and if you would like further information we can continue now or at a later time. We need to make the local coroner's office aware of the death as it was unexpected. They will then make the decision as to whether a post-mortem examination is required, which will be done in consultation with you. We will put you in touch with the Bereavement services here who will be able to guide you."

66 **Relatives:** *"Will we be able to see him before all of this?"*

You: "You will be able to see him shortly. We will move him from theatres to a quiet room where you can spend some time with him."

COMMUNICATION

How do you close the consultation?

It is important to leave support in place after the consultation and to arrange the next point of contact, as there will be further questions once they are over the initial shock. Ask whether the family would like to have the Nurse stay with them or whether they would like a moment alone. Offer to come back at a later time to answer any further questions and give contact details for Bereavement Services.

You: "I'm sure you would like some time alone as a family. Would you like the nurse to stay with you?"

66 **Relatives:** *"No thank you, we would like to have some time alone."*

You: "Take as much time as you need. I will come back later to answer any further questions you may have. The Nurses are on the ward should you need anything in the meantime. Do you have any further questions for me now?"

66 **Relatives:** *"You're the junior doctor aren't you? Can we speak to the Consultant?"*

You: "Of course. Miss Banks is still in theatres and will be down shortly to see you."

66 **Relative:** *"Thank you Doctor."*

✎ Comm Skills Tip: Dealing With Grief and Anger

Some people express grief in this situation by anger and aggressive behaviour. In this scenario there are a few things to remember:

- If there is physical aggression directed at you then the best thing is to try to defuse the situation if you feel able. If it becomes apparent that you cannot, you should take the safest course of action which would be for you and the Nurse to leave and return at a later time. This will almost certainly not be the case in the exam (they won't want you walking out of the exam station!) so if the patient becomes angry it is likely that you will have to defuse the situation.
- Allow the relative to talk and shout if they need to. Remain passive and seated and do not match the relative's body language. By remaining seated you encourage them to re-take their seat when they start to calm down. Keep your own body language open.
- If the relatives are angry you need to be careful how you phrase your statements so that you do not come across as inflammatory, patronising or uncaring as this will exacerbate the situation. Take a moment to think before you speak.
- Don't interrupt.

You: "I understand that this is a very emotional time for you and your family. Please take a seat and I can try to answer your questions" [give them the opportunity to continue the consultation]

You: "If you'd like I can come back in a little while and answer your questions."

SUMMARY

This can feel like some of the most difficult bad news to tell someone. The reaction to the news cannot easily be anticipated. Some people may cry, some may become angry and some may say nothing at all. You need to be prepared for any eventuality.

Deliver the news in a calm and solemn manner. You can use phrases like 'has passed away' and 'did not make it'. Saying that a relative 'has died' can feel harsh although it would not be inappropriate. 'Has not survived' is a nice phrase to use as it is still clinical but does not sound cold. Whichever way you choose to word it, practice saying it to others in mock scenarios and find what feels best for you. Often you will not get past saying "I'm sorry…" before you get a reaction from the family.

Follow up with information as it is asked for. Leave a respectful period of silence after breaking the news. The consultation will then be led by the relatives, ether they will initiate questions or you may have to suggest that they may have questions. Answer questions simply and without being verbose. As always, be honest and if you cannot answer a question either signpost or offer to find out and come back.
It is important to signpost to the Bereavement Services at the hospital as part of 'what will happen next'. Bereavement Services provide information and support for relatives in these situations.

Actor Brief

Alison Shardlow is the wife (or daughter) of Peter Shardlowa 66 yearol-old gentleman. You are aware that Peter was admitted as an emergency overnight. The A&E doctor mentioned an aneurysm and that it was quite serious. You spoke briefly with the surgical team and understand that it was a big operation. Peter was otherwise well and you are a close family.

Special Instructions: The actor should be very upset on hearing the news. Silence and crying as appropriate. The actor should prompt by asking about post-mortems and about the bereavement process.

TOP TIPS

Always keep your body language passive and open. Sit slightly bent forward, don't fold arms or legs, hold your hands loosely in front of you. Your role is to be supportive and to answer questions. Keep your language simple and caring, remember not to be patronising or blunt.

The latter part of this consultation will involve you sign posting to Bereavement Services and, if the family wish, to the Patient Liaison Services for example if they wish to make a complaint. The scenario will focus on how you deliver the news and your interaction with the actor, and with how you practically deal with answering questions and giving guidance as to the next steps.

COMMUNICATION

2.3 | Colonic Cancer Biopsy Result

Scenario

You are the CT2 in clinic and your next patient is Mr. Jenkins. He is a 64-year-old ex-smoker with a background of mild COPD and a myocardial infarction 10 years ago. He was initially referred by his GP with a history of weight loss and blood in the stool. He has had a colonoscopy and biopsy. The histology report from the biopsy has returned as moderately differentiated adenocarcinoma. He has returned to clinic for his biopsy results.

You have washed your hands and introduced yourself. Please tell the patient the results of his biopsy.

How would you open the consultation?

Establish what the patient understands so far and that they are expecting the biopsy results. You can ask them to briefly recap the history and quickly establish some concerns (cancer) and expectations (possible bad news). This should be done briefly as the patient will understandably be anxious and has come today to be given the results, so try not to stall giving the news.

You: "I've read through your notes but please could you briefly tell me in your own words what has been happening over the last few months?"

66 **Patient:** *"OK Doctor, yes, I went to see my GP about two months ago as I'd been losing weight and had noticed some blood when I went to the toilet. My GP sent me to this clinic and they arranged for me to have the camera test. During the test they saw something unusual so they took a piece to send off to the lab. I was told to come back today to get the results."*

How would you continue?

You: "So today you're expecting your biopsy results. Is there anyone with you who you'd like to bring in for the consultation?" [first warning shot]

66 **Patient:** *"No, my wife is at work, I've come on my own."*

You: "Do you have any particular ideas or concerns about the biopsy?" [second warning shot]

66 **Patient:** *"Yes, of course, I mean, blood in the motion and what with me being a smoker for so many years, I'm really worried it's cancer. Do you have the results?"*

How would you deliver the bad news?

It is best to be straight with the patient. Don't shy away from using the word 'cancer' as it will leave no doubt or question as to the diagnosis. After telling the news, give a period of silence to let the news sink in.

You: "I'm sorry to have to tell you that the results do show a cancer in the bowel." At this point pause to allow the patient to process the news.

What do you do next?

The patient may have an emotional response to the news, or not know what to say. If the patient cries, offer them a tissue. Keep body language open and supportive. The patient may continue the consultation and ask for further information. If the patient does not speak after a pause you can continue to deliver more information as it is important to reassure that there are steps that can be taken and that this cancer is potentially curable.

> 66 **Patient:** *"So, is that it for me doc? Am I done for? Is there anything that can be done?"*

You: "I understand that you will have a lot of questions. Firstly I want to reassure you that the majority of cancers of the bowel are very treatable. This is usually with a combination of chemotherapy and surgery. Before we make plans for treatment we will need to do further scans to see if the cancer has spread anywhere. Once we have the scans we will discuss your case at a meeting between the surgeons, the Radiology doctors and the Oncology doctors and we will determine the best way to tailor your treatment to you."

How will you answer the patient's questions?

The patient may have a variety of questions but these would be some typical ones to anticipate. Do your best to answer all of their questions as best you can in an honest and open way. You can give some reassurance that there are treatment options and cure is a possibility. Remember to be clear that treatment will depend on the MDT outcome and that support is available through Specialist Nurses/ Macmillan Nurses.

> 66 **Patient:** *"So you can do something? That's a relief. I have so many questions. Will I need surgery?"*

You: "These cancers often require surgery, which can usually remove all of the tumour"

> 66 **Patient:** *"Will I be left with a bag? An uncle of mine had a bag after having cancer of the bowel"*

You: "You may or may not require a stoma as part of the surgery, which is a bag stuck onto your belly to collect your motions. These are sometimes permanent but often we can re-plumb things inside at a later operation to remove the need for the bag. If we are considering a stoma we will put you in touch with our Stoma Specialist Nurses who will be able to give you lots of information about living with a stoma and how to minimise the impact on your daily life."

> 66 **Patient:** *"If I need chemotherapy will I have to take a lot of time off work? I'm self-employed and need to work to put food on the table."*

You: "You will need to take time to recuperate after any surgery and often chemotherapy can make you feel quite unwell. People respond differently and some people need to take more time off than others. There are avenues available for support, both with finances and everyday living. We have Specialist Nurses in the hospital who will be able to help with all of these concerns as they arise."

COMMUNICATION

How will you continue the consultation?

Signpost the next steps and make sure there are no outstanding questions.

You: "So the next thing to do is for me to arrange for you to have some scans. We will write to you with the appointments for those. In the mean time I would like to put you in touch with our Specialist Nurse who will be able to help you with any further questions you may have, and be a point of contact for you. Do you have any more questions for me?"

❝ Patient: *"No, I can't think of any more questions at the moment."*

How do you close the consultation?

How and when the consultation is closed will depend on the patient. Make sure that you have answered all of their questions. In these scenarios the actor will guide you, if there is something you have missed they will ask/allude to it more than once, but if you fail to spot it they will not press the issue. Be mindful if the actor is repeating something as it is almost certainly a hint!

You: "OK, we will see you back in clinic again in two weeks after we have discussed your scans and biopsy result at our big meeting. We can then talk about how we are going to proceed. In the mean time I will ask our Specialist Nurse to contact you and I will also make sure we have an up to date contact number for you."

❝ Patient: *"OK, thank you Doctor. I'll wait for my next scan appointment in the post. This is my best contact number, I'll wait for the nurse to call."*

SUMMARY

In this scenario it is important to be open and honest in how the news is delivered but you can also give the patient some reassurance, as adenocarcinoma of the colon is often very treatable. Do not offer false reassurance as we do not yet have information about the extent of the tumour or metastases.
Deliver news about a cancer diagnosis early in the consultation as the patient has come expecting their results and will often be anxious to have their fears either confirmed or dismissed.

Allow some pauses as these will allow the patient to gather their thoughts. They may have many or few questions. Encourage the patient to ask questions and if they need time to think allow this. Reassure the patient that if they think of further questions after the consultation they have a point of contact.
Be clear as to the next steps. You will organise a scan and they will hear from you, and treatment decisions will be made on the basis of a few more investigations and MDT discussion.

TOP TIPS

➕ Remember the importance of body language in these scenarios. You will both likely to be sat facing each other in a clinic setting. The set-up will likely already have you facing each other but try to avoid being across a desk from the patient. Keep your demeanor open and supportive.

➕ You can offer some reassurance in this scenario as there are good treatment options available, but don't be falsely reassuring. Never use absolutes! You should only speak in terms of likelihood.

➕ Getting other team members involved in this scenario is imperative. Mention the MDT and introduce the Specialist Nurse. In the scenario it is unlikely there will be a 'Specialist Nurse' actor in with you, as opposed to in clinic where they would accompany you for the consultation, so make plans for the patient to be contacted.

😐 Actor Brief

You are Mr./Mrs. Halden. You have previously been fit and well but in the last 4 or 5 months you have noticed that you are intermittently constipated. You do also occasionally have some diarrhoea. You have also noticed some bright red blood on the toilet paper, which is worrying you a lot.

You think you have maybe lost a bit of weight over the same period – you are reasonably active so think it may be just due to that. You have lost about half a stone. Your energy levels are normal.

You have no abdominal pain that you have noticed. You are not nauseated. You have no urinary or gynaecological symptoms.

PMH: Open appendicectomy aged 15.

DH: Allergic to penicillin. No regular medications.

FH: Mother has diverticular disease. Father died of heart attack aged 66.

SH: You drink 3-4 glasses of wine a week. You are an ex-smoker – you smoked 10 cigarettes a day for about 10 years, quitting 40 years ago. You are a retired secretary. You live independently with your husband/wife.

Systems Review: Nil else of note

COMMUNICATION

2.4 | Explaining DNAR

Scenario

You are the CT2 on the ward. During the night Mrs. Saunders was admitted with acute bowel obstruction. She is 83 years old and very frail, with a background of ischaemic heart disease, hypertension and a laparotomy twenty years ago for bowel cancer, which was treated successfully. She lives in warden supported accommodation with frequent visits by her son. She is being treated with intravenous fluids and a naso-gastric tube on a provisional diagnosis of adhesional bowel obstruction. She is currently stable and will have a CT scan later today.

The Consultant Mr. Sparks has suggested that a DNAR form would be appropriate for this patient. He has asked you to discuss the form with Mrs. Saunder's son who is next of kin. Mrs. Saunders has given permission for you to speak to her son. You have washed your hands and introduced yourself.

How would you open the consultation?

It is important to gain good rapport from the outset. The DNAR form is designed to prevent unnecessary suffering and it is important that the family have a shared understanding of why we implement them, what they mean and their limitations.
It is always good to open a consultation by ascertaining what the other person knows and understands so far and gauge their expectations.

You: "Good afternoon Mr. Saunders. I've been asked to speak to you by Mr. Sparks, the Consultant looking after your mother. Can you tell me what you understand so far?"

❝ **Relative:** *"Well, I know Mum is very ill at the moment. She has not been herself for a couple of months and last night she just got very sick so the warden called an ambulance which brought her here. The night doctor told me that there is a blockage in her bowel, which obviously worried me as she had bowel cancer many years ago. She had an operation at the time, which cured it, but I'm concerned it could have come back. She's not as fit as she used to be and I'm really worried for her."*

How would you introduce the concept of DNAR?

It can be difficult to broach the subject of DNAR. A good way to test the water is to enquire as to whether the patient themselves had ever expressed any wishes relating to CPR. This should also reveal whether the patient has an advanced directive or community DNAR.

You: "I understand your concern. We plan to do a CT scan later today to get to the bottom of what has caused her to be unwell. Whilst you mum is on the ward with us, we need to speak to you about whether she had ever expressed any feelings about having resuscitation should her heart stop."

❝ **Relative:** *"Like doing chest compressions? I'm sure she spoke about this with the doctors when she was in with her bowel cancer years ago, but I can't remember* *if she had any strong feelings. Surely whilst she's in hospital you'd do everything you could to help her?"*

How would you continue the consultation?

This is a perfect opportunity for you to explain the difference between not treating a patient and opting not to perform CPR due to perceived futility. You can explain that everything else will be done to diagnose and treat what is wrong but should cardiac arrest occur we would not do CPR as this would not fix the underlying problem and could cause unnecessary suffering.

You: "We will continue to actively treat your mum and what we do next will depend on what we find on the CT scan. What we need to discuss is what we should do in the event of a cardiac arrest, meaning that if her heart were to stop unexpectedly and cause sudden death." [removes doubt]

❝❝ Relative: *"So you are still going to do the scan and give her treatment?"*

You: "Yes."

❝❝ Relative: *"But if her heart stops you don't want to try and save her?"*

You: "If the heart stops this causes death. Doing chest compressions does not fix the underlying cause of the heart stopping. If we were to give CPR this involves heavy chest compressions, which break ribs. It can be very traumatic. It can be a very undignified and unpleasant way to pass away." [causing harm/ perpetuating suffering/ lack of dignity in death]

How would you deal with the following?

❝❝ Relative: *"It sounds like you're writing her off!"*

You: "I want to reassure you that we plan to continue investigating and treating her illness as we would any other patient. The reason we talk about CPR is for if the unexpected happens. Some people express wishes that they do not want to be resuscitated and some people have agreements in the community that mean their wishes are honoured.
It is important also to explain from our medical point of view when we do not think something will be in someone's best interests. In this case we believe that should the unexpected happen, performing CPR would cause more harm than it would do any good."

Continue to answer the relative's questions

❝❝ Relative: *"So is it up to me whether you do CPR or not?"*

You: "Whether to do CPR is always a medical decision that will be made by the doctors, so don't feel pressured that this decision rests with you. When we are considering putting a 'Do Not Resuscitate' form in place we always discuss with the patient if they are able, anyone with power of attorney, and the next of kin. If the patient does not want CPR they can tell us. If we do not think CPR would work we can explain this. We let the family know about these decisions so that everyone is fully informed."

COMMUNICATION

66 **Relative:** *"If you sign this form does it stay with her even if she gets better?"*

You: "The decision is dynamic and we review it every day. As a patient's condition changes the decision may no longer be appropriate in which case we can cancel the form. If someone has a decision made in the community, for example with the GP, we still always review it when they come into hospital. Similarly when she leaves hospital the 'Do Not Resuscitate' form will not go with her. If she is to come into hospital again at a later time the form will not be valid and a new one would have to be considered if appropriate."

How would you draw the consultation to a close?

You: "Do you have any further concerns about the DNAR form?"

66 **Relative:** *"Well, I understand everything you have explained so far. I understand that this is a decision by the Doctors but I want to make sure Mum gets the best care. If she were to suddenly get very ill I want her to still be treated."*

You: "If she were to become more ill we would continue to treat as we would anyone else. The DNAR form is purely in the event of death, about whether we do chest compressions. In this case we feel that chest compressions would be futile and would contribute to an undignified death."

66 **Relative:** *"OK, I understand. Please help Mum as best you can. If she were to die unexpectedly I would want her to go peacefully."*

How would you finish the consultation?

Ensure the relative has no further questions. The actor in the scenario will always guide you so listen carefully to everything they say. If they repeat questions this is a hint.

You: "Do you have any further questions?"

66 **Relative:** *"No. Thank you for taking the time to explain."*

You: "If you think of anything further that you would like to clarify, the nursing staff on the ward know how to contact me and I'm happy to speak with you again."

SUMMARY

We all know that a DNAR decision is purely a medical one and a family cannot make a decision as to whether or not to have one. A patient is within their rights to refuse CPR if they have capacity to make decisions and may well have an advanced directive in place. That being said it is best practice to involve both the patient and the family in DNAR decisions to establish whether they have strong feelings.

The DNAR decision should be first and foremost discussed with the patient. The patient can decline to discuss it or may not be competent to discuss it e.g. if reduced GCS. A patient can request not to have CPR, even if it would be appropriate.

There are lots of things in this scenario to discuss and lots of opportunity for questions from the relative/patient. It is possible that the actor in this scenario could become angry or upset so be prepared for this. If you have a good starting point for the conversation and have thought ahead about how you would broach the subject often it can be done without

the scenario escalating. It is important to build rapport early in the scenario.
You may find yourself talking a lot during this scenario as there is a lot for you to explain.
Remember to leave appropriate breaks in the conversation to allow questioning and
encourage questions at the end.

☺ **Actor Brief**

Michael Saunders is a 53-year-old partner at a law firm. You understand that
your mother has been quite unwell and are worried as she is already quite frail.
You have been told by the doctors that your mother has a bowel obstruction. You
are not from a medical background and are not sure how serious this might be.

Special Instructions: When first discussing DNAR you are concerned that the
doctors are giving up and you may wish to become angry.

TOP TIPS

➕ Be very factual in how you speak. Try to refer to 'death' rather
than 'the heart stopping' or 'cardiac arrest' as this leaves no doubt
about when and why we do CPR.

➕ Be explicit that a DNAR decision is NOT a decision not to treat.

➕ Remember in real life if you need advice you can always defer to
your defence union at any time of day or night and the hospital
palliative care team are a helpful source of information.

COMMUNICATION

2.5 Paediatric Appendicectomy

Scenario

Jack Williams is a 10-year-old who has been diagnosed with acute appendicitis and admitted to the Paediatric ward. It is 6pm and the consultant on call, Ms. Griggs, is planning to take him to theatre later this evening once the current laparotomy is finished. Ms. Griggs has asked you to consent him as she is in theatre. He is currently stable but pyrexial at 37.8 degrees Celsius. He is otherwise fit and well. His mother Mrs. Williams is present at the bedside.

You have washed your hands and introduced yourself. A history and examination have been performed. Please consent this child for an appendicectomy.

How would you begin?

You: "Hello Jack, I'm Dr. X, one of the surgeons here this evening. And who's here with you?"

66 **Patient:** *"That's my mum."*

You: "Hello Mrs. Williams, my consultant Ms. Griggs has asked me to come and discuss what we are planning to do next and to answer any questions you may have. Can I just check what you've been told so far?"

66 **Mother:** *"Why hasn't the consultant come to talk to me? I've been told Jack needs an operation this evening! Why am I having to talk to a junior?"*

You: "Mrs. Williams, I'm sorry the consultant cannot be here at this moment. I've come to talk to you about Jack's appendicitis at her request. Ms. Griggs is Jack's consultant but unfortunately she is currently operating on another very sick patient. She felt it best for Jack if I discussed the operation with you now and then if you were happy to proceed you could sign the consent form. In turn this would then mean there would be no delay in him being treated."

66 **Mother:** *"OK. But will the consultant be doing the procedure?"*

You: "I believe so but I cannot guarantee it. If it is not her, it will be someone senior who is experienced and knows what they are doing"

66 **Mother:** *"OK."* (Settles down and is more open/helpful at this point if she is reassured)

What will you ask next?

You: "Before I explain the operation it would be helpful to know what you've already been told?"

Mother: *"Well the paediatric doctor said that Jack would be having an operation. That his appendix was infected or something. But that's all I was told. The next thing the nurse was telling me this operation would be tonight!"*

You: "I understand that must have come as a bit of a shock. Appendicitis is the inflammation and infection of a small extension of the bowel that is found in the right lower part of the abdomen. It does not have any function but can become inflamed. When this happens it can cause pain and make the person unwell. It is a very common condition and we often can delay surgery until the following day. However if someone is particularly unwell or if we are worried the appendix might burst or has burst then we try to operate sooner. In Jack's case I don't think his appendix has burst yet but it is at risk of doing so."

Mother: *"Ah. That makes more sense, that must be why he's so unwell and in so much pain."*

What will you ask next?

You: "I will go through the risks and benefits of the operation but before I do is there anything in particular that's worrying you or that you would like to ask?"

Mother: *"Will Jack be asleep for this? I'm worried about him being scared, and how long the procedure will take."*

You: "I understand, it can be a lot to take in when you've just been told someone you care about needs surgery. Jack will be anaesthetised (put to sleep) for the operation. The anaesthetist will go through the details with you before he is taken to the operating theatre. You'll be able to come down to the anaesthetic room with him so he won't be alone. The procedure takes approximately 35-45 minutes although it can be longer and it can be shorter. I'm sorry I cannot be more specific than that."

Explain the procedure?

You: "The procedure itself can be performed by keyhole surgery or by making a larger cut over the area of the appendix on the right side of the tummy. In children we often perform an open procedure as the size and number of keyholes we need end up being larger than one small cut. In either case we will identify the appendix, tie it off and remove it. It can be removed via a keyhole or via the open cut made. Sometimes even when we start with a keyhole procedure we have to abandon it and convert the procedure to an open procedure. If this has happened it is because we could not deal with the appendix via the keyholes or if there were also abscesses that needed draining."

Mother: *"OK, I understand. Hopefully it won't come to that."*

Explain the risks and benefits of the procedure

You: "The benefits of the operation are to prevent worsening infection, remove the appendix and improve pain. I need to tell you about all the serious risks that can occur. We do everything we can to minimise the risks involved but complications do occur. The main general risks are bleeding, infection and anaesthetic risks. There is a theoretical risk of clots in the legs or lungs but in someone young and generally healthy this is very unlikely. Specific risks of this operation are damage to the bowel or bladder, converting the keyhole

COMMUNICATION

procedure into an open procedure, hernia and scarring in the abdomen called adhesions. Sometimes the appendix we take out looks normal, in which case the appendix was probably not the cause. In some cases we never know what exactly was causing the pain but if we have ruled out all serious possibilities, such as appendicitis, then we can safely assume it was something simple and not serious after all. If this happens but Jack improves then we can let him go home in a day or two after the operation. In Jack's case, because of his symptoms it is very likely this is appendicitis. Do you have any questions?"

❝ **Mother:** *"OK. I understand. No I think you've covered everything. Oh no, I meant to ask, what happens after? He loves playing rugby and has a match soon."*

Explain what recovery entails

You: "After the operation we'll keep Jack in hospital until he starts to show signs of improvement and that the pain is under control. This usually takes a day or two. If he is well and not having any further temperatures or worsening tummy pain then we'll be able to let him go home. He'll be able to go back to playing sports in 2-3 weeks."

❝ **Mother:** *"Thank you doctor."*

How would you close the consultation?

You: "No problem Mrs. Williams. I've explained the risks and benefits of the operation to remove the appendix which we believe is inflamed and infected in Jack's case. I've also explained what to expect after he returns from theatre. Hopefully now it's much clearer about what will happen. The anaesthetist will be along shortly to discuss the anaesthetic plans with you. If you are happy to proceed I will need you to sign the consent form, which outlines what we have discussed. "

SUMMARY

Appendicitis is a common condition (roughly 1 in 13 will develop it during their lifetime) that affects both children and adults but most commonly between 10-20 years old. There is a second peak incidence in patients in their seventies.

In general pain precedes vomiting and cases usually present with a low grade fever (<38). While many cases present with the textbook umbilical pain that then moves to the right iliac fossa, this does not always occur and may present with pain in the RUQ/suprapubic region depending on the lie of the appendix.

In consenting for an appendicectomy remember to mention that sometimes the appendix is normal and that a definite diagnosis cannot always be given for the cause of abdominal pain.

☺ **Actor Brief**

You (Mrs. Williams – patient's mother) are a protective knowledgeable mother who works as a primary school teacher.

General information: You are initially angry that a 'junior' surgeon is coming to talk to you but if the doctor explains early on that Ms. Griggs is operating and is unable to come and that this is the best way to ensure your son receives urgent surgery you settle and become attentive and less demanding.

Presenting Complaint: Jack had 2-3 days going off his food, developing tummy ache and then more severe pain then started vomiting. At first you thought it was a 'tummy bug' but when he became feverish and still wasn't eating/drinking you came to the Emergency Department.

ICE: You are expecting a consultant to come see you. Once the doctor explains that a consultant is around and that the procedure will happen tonight you settle.

Significant PMH/DH/SH: eczema, NKDA, non-smoking household (rest of family are well)

Special Instructions: If the doctor does not appropriately (ie with understanding/empathy and reassurance) explain that the consultant is around for the procedure but cannot do the consent you can become demanding about seeing someone senior until the doctor reassures you that this is the best course for getting your son's operation organised quickly.

TOP TIPS

✚ ALWAYS check who is bedside with a minor. Never assume it is the mother/father/legal guardian. If the child is old enough, an easy way to develop rapport is to first address the child and ask who the other person is. Otherwise check with staff.

✚ Patients/relatives will often ask if the consultant is the one operating. We all know that it is sometimes the registrar/SHO who will actually do the procedure +/- under supervision. Ultimately do not lie and if you are too vague on who is doing the procedure the patient/relative will pick up on this. Stick to saying that you cannot guarantee who is doing the procedure as you will not necessarily be in the operating theatre at the time of the operation but that the procedure will be performed by someone who knows what they are doing (this is actually listed on all consent forms!).

COMMUNICATION

2.6 | Consent: ERCP

Scenario

Ms. Barnaby is a 56-year-old lady admitted from the surgical assessment unit with right upper quadrant pain, deranged LFTs and a known diagnosis of gallstones. She has a simple past medical history of hypertension only. You are seeing her on the ward and the consultant has asked you to consent her for an ERCP later today. You have washed your hands and introduced yourself.

Please consent this patient for an ERCP.

How would you begin?

You: "Ms. Barnaby? Hello, I'm Dr. X. I've come to talk to you about the risks and benefits of a procedure called an ERCP that we think you need to help with the gallstones. Can you tell me what you've been told so far?"

Patient: "Well I've been told that one of my gallstones is blocking the tube that lets, is it bile?, Go into the stomach and that it needs to be unblocked, or something?"

What will you ask next?

Establish any ideas, concerns or expectations that the patient may have and then signpost that you will explain the risks and benefits of the procedure.

You: "Exactly. Did anyone explain how this would be done?"

Patient: "No"

You: "I'd like to explain the details of how we do an ERCP but before I do is there anything you are particularly worried about?"

Patient: "Honestly doctor I don't want to be in pain, will this procedure hurt at all?"

You: "I understand your worry, generally this procedure is well tolerated but there's always a risk of complications. I'd like to explain what an ERCP entails and then I'll go on to explain all the major risks associated with it. Lastly we can talk about pain and what can be done if you do experience pain and I'll answer any further questions you may have. If you're happy to go ahead with this I'll then ask you to sign the consent form"

Patient: "OK"

You: "So as we've discussed, a gallstone is blocking the tube, the common bile duct, that allows bile to drain from the liver into the intestines. This is causing the pain and the problem with your liver enzymes. In order to unblock this we would like to use a thin camera, which goes down your throat into your tummy and can find the tube that is blocked. At this point we use a dye which allows us to see where the blockage is and at the same time we can try to fish out the stone or stones which are causing the problem."

Patient: "What if you can't fish out the stones?"

You: "Sometimes we can stretch the tube or make a tiny nick in the opening of the tube to allow bigger stones to come out. Occasionally we have to leave a drain in the tube if we cannot get the stone out. This allows the bile to get past the blockage. In these cases we'd then come back in 4-6 weeks to take the drain out and try to remove the remaining stone. Alternatively we might then need to consider operating on your tummy and removing your gallbladder and exploring the tube to find the blockage."

66 **Patient:** "OK. So first we try this ERCP you've mentioned?"

You: "Yes. Now the main benefits of this procedure are to diagnose the blockage – so to understand where the tube is blocked and how, to remove the gallstones, to prevent problems developing with your liver as a result of the blockage and to reduce the risk of infection. The main risks are divided into general risks and risks specific to this procedure. General risks include infection, bleeding, breathing or heart problems, anaesthetic risks and clots developing in your legs or lungs. The specific risks include pancreatitis (this is where your pancreas becomes inflamed and painful) and this is relatively common. 1 in 20 to 1 in 10 develop this complication. Other risks include bowel injury, bile duct (tube) injury and failure to remove the gallstones as I've explained. Do you have any questions?"

66 **Patient:** "What happens if I get this problem with my pancreas?"

You: "In the first instance we give you pain killers and lots of fluids via a drip. We also monitor your blood tests regularly. In most cases this is all that's needed."

66 **Patient:** "OK I'm happy to sign the consent form then."

How would you close the consultation?

You: "Ms. Barnaby, just to recap what we've discussed: We'll be scheduling you for an ERCP which is a camera test which allows us to identify the blockage from the gallstone (s) and attempt to remove it. I've discussed the benefits and risks and you've signed the consent form. If you experience any pain we will make sure you have pain killers available to control the pain. Thank you."

66 **Patient:** "OK thank you Doctor."

COMMUNICATION

SUMMARY

Gallstones causing CBD dilatation and obstruction are common and ERCP is often the first line modality to treat a patient with an acute obstructive picture and abdominal pain. Pancreatitis is a common serious complication and as such needs to be appropriately explained.

Patients with gallstones can be stratified into low, intermediate and high risk patients. Low risk patients should be listed for a laparoscopic (+/-open) cholecystectomy. Intermediate risk patients (identified by mildly abnormal LFTs, previous pancreatitis/cholangitis or dilated CBD 8-10mm) should have further imaging e.g. MRCP or USS before further management is planned. High risk patients should be listed for ERCP. This group includes recent acute pancreatitis/cholangitis, jaundice, abnormal LFTs (ALP higher than double the normal value) and/or a CBD >10mm.

☺ **Actor Brief**

You are a 56-year-old overweight anxious lady with no husband or partner. You are anxious, in pain (although this is about 6/10 at present) and you feel vulnerable at being on your own in hospital.

Presenting Complaint: You've had several episodes of RUQ pain over the past few months after eating, it previously settled with co-codamol bought over the counter. You've been trying to lose weight and have been successful in losing 1 stone (6.3kg) over the past 3 months with a weight watching group. You were admitted via ambulance yesterday when after an episode of RUQ pain lasted >1 hour and pain was 10/10 with nausea. Blood tests showed an obstructive cholestatic picture and ultrasound showed a dilated CBD (common bile duct) suggesting blockage with a gallstone. You understand you have a gallstone stuck.

ICE: You are very afraid of being in pain and have unrealistic expectations of what pain killers/doctors can achieve.

PMH/DH/SH: Hypertension. Overweight. Allergic to dogs and plasters. Ex-smoker quit 20 years ago. Live alone in a flat, work as a cook in a school kitchen.

Special Instructions: You are unrealistic about pain – you believe there must be some magic fix that is risk free that can guarantee no pain – be persistent in asking if the doctor can promise you a pain free procedure unless they appropriately explain that it is impossible to guarantee this but that there will be good pain relief available.

TOP TIPS

✚ This is a commonly performed procedure but pancreatitis is quite a common complication *(~1 in 10)* and in this patient she is clearly afraid of being in pain. Make sure you reassure her but do not downplay the likelihood of post-ERCP pain

✚ Make sure the patient knows it is not always possible to get all the gallstones out and that they may need repeat procedures!

2.7 | Fractured Neck Of Femur

Scenario

Mrs. Tibbet is an 81-year-old patient who suffers with dementia. She was admitted to the trauma ward following a fall in her care home and has been found to have an intracapsular neck of femur fracture. Her daughter has come in to find out what has happened and what will happen next.

You have washed your hands and introduced yourself. Please explain to the patient's daughter what has happened and what will happen next.

How would you begin?

You: "Good evening Miss Tibbet. I'm Dr. X. Your mother has been admitted to this ward following a fall. Before I begin answering any questions you might have I'd like to find out what you've been told so far please."

66 **Relative:** "The care home called me, they said mother had been a bit more confused overnight and when they came in at 6am they found her on the floor unable to move her left leg. The doctors in A&E said that she'd broken her hip. I'm so worried!"

You: "I understand. And how much do you know about what happens when someone breaks their hip?"

66 **Relative:** "Well I know she broke her wrist a year ago, they just put it in a cast and it healed up. Does this work the same way?"

You: "Unfortunately not. The x-ray confirmed a break at the top of her leg in her hip joint. If left alone it is very unlikely to heal and she will struggle to ever walk on her leg again. If a patient is well enough we usually recommend surgery".

66 **Relative:** "Oh no! I can't believe this is happening! First her wrist, now this!"

What will you ask next?

You: "Is there anything in particular you're worried about before we discuss what happens next?"

66 **Relative:** "Well this is so sudden. I'm so upset. Some of the staff in the care home are really rude, I can't believe they left her all night on the floor. They're supposed to check on her overnight because she does tend to wander about! Will she die?"

You: "It is a rather serious injury and in someone with many other health issues, the risks including death or other complications does increase but this is a very common injury and there are well established options for treating a broken hip - the majority of people do reasonably well. You mentioned you have concerns about the care home staff, I will try to find out exactly what happened. If I find anything that sounds inappropriate I will raise it with my seniors"

COMMUNICATION

66 **Relative:** "Oh thank you"

(There are potential safety issues here as well as the relative's concerns. Do not ignore this but do not get focused on that aspect for this station.)

Explain what the procedure involves

You: "When someone breaks their hip in the way that your mother has, we are faced with two surgical options. We can replace the ball and the socket of the hip joint or we can replace just the ball of the hip joint leaving the patient's own hip socket intact. I understand she fell overnight but has she had any other falls recently?"

66 **Relative:** "Well, she's been a bit more unsteady over the past couple of years but I put that down to her getting on a bit. She now uses a walking frame all the time."

You: "In someone who already has limited mobility, such as your mother, replacing just the ball of the hip works well. We use a metal implant shaped like the hip joint."

66 **Relative:** "That sounds very extreme. Does she definitely need an operation?"

Explain the reasons for doing the procedure

You: "As I mentioned, if left alone, she is very unlikely to ever be able to walk again. When we are unable to fix a broken hip, patients are often bedridden. This can lead to other problems such as chest infections and bed sores. Unfortunately there is no easy option and we need to find the best option for your mother that balances the benefits against any risks."

66 **Relative:** "I see. It sounds as though she really should have the operation. What will it allow her to do?"

Explain the procedure and recovery

You: "The procedure I am proposing is called a Hemiarthroplasty. This means a half hip joint. As I started to explain, we would remove the broken top bit of the hip where the ball is and replace that with a metal ball on a long stem which then acts as the main part of the hip joint and sits in the hip socket. This would allow her to get back on her feet. This could be as early as the same or next day as the operation although it does take weeks for a patient to recover fully. She'd be seen by the physiotherapists to help with this."

66 **Relative:** "What can go wrong?"

Explain the risks associated with this procedure

You: "Well there are general risks associated with surgery and then there are risks specific to this operation. We do what we can to minimise these risks and they are not common however I do need to explain them to you so you understand what complications can occur.
There are risks such as bleeding, so much so that your mother needs a transfusion. Infection is also a risk, we give antibiotics at the time of surgery to help prevent infection. There are also anaesthetic risks. The anaesthetist will go through the specifics of those risks with you and your mother before the operation. There is also a risk of clots in the legs and even in the lungs. If clot travels to the lungs it can be fatal. With this particular operation

there is a risk of leg length differences, breaking the bone when the new hip is put in and there's also a risk that the implant fails - although this is rare."

66   **Relative:** "Oh doctor there's a lot that can go wrong! Could she die?"

You: "Unfortunately that is a possibility, but we will do everything we can to reduce the risk of that happening."

How would you close the consultation?

You: "Miss Tibbet, your mother had a fall overnight and broke her left hip. She ideally needs an operation to fix this as I have explained. Do you have any questions or would you like anything clarified?"

66   **Relative**: "Thank you no, I think you've explained everything."

SUMMARY

In explaining a hip fracture to a relative or indeed the patient themselves you should ensure you first establish what they know/have been told. It's simple but checking that they know their hip is broken is important. You'd be surprised how often it's not been mentioned what the x-ray showed. Going through the need for surgery and the risks versus benefits is especially important in this case as the patient is usually frail and often has many comorbidities which affect overall mortality. Neck of femur fracture patients have high mortality rates: 10% die in hospital within 1 month and 30% are dead at 1 year. This needs to be explained in a balanced way to patients and their families. Also try to include what happens after surgery as this is often what people worry about – when will they walk again? How soon can they leave hospital?

😐 **Actor brief**

You are an anxious 52-year-old woman who is very concerned for her mother and are having this discussion in the relative's room in the Emergency Department at 4:45am.

You are already angry and upset that the care home 'let' your mother fall and you have previous grievances with the care home manager about standard of care, which are influencing your current mood. You are keen for your mother to avoid surgery

Presenting Complaint: The patient Mrs. Tibbet suffers with severe dementia and has developed a UTI, which has increased her confusion resulting in increased nocturia. As a result of this last night she has lost her balance and fallen.

ICE: Mrs. Tibbet has previously told you that if it's her time to go she wants doctors to let her go. You understand and support your mother in these wishes. You are worried about your mother dying but also about your mother being able to walk again.

COMMUNICATION

PMH/DH/SH: Mrs. Tibbet suffers with dementia, osteoporosis, COPD and has previously had a CVA. She has broken her wrist recently. She has NKDA and has so many medications you can't remember them. She used to smoke 15/day. She lives in a care home and uses a zimmer frame.

Special Instructions: If the risk of death is reeled off without some attempt at easing the information into the conversation you become hysterical and start crying.

TOP TIPS

➕ Make sure to use words like ball and socket that the lay person will understand.

➕ If you have paper, drawings in this kind of explanation of surgery are very useful.

➕ Do not shirk from the honest answer when a patient/relative asks if someone could die during surgery.

➕ Although the patient suffers with severe dementia, she may still have previously expressed wishes about resuscitation. This may also be explored if you have time.

2.8 | Consent For A Trial

Scenario

You are the Urology SHO and have assisted your consultant in setting up a trial. He has just seen Mr.. Smith in clinic who he feels would be suitable and has asked you to consent him for enrolment in the trial. He has already been consented for the specific procedure.

In this station you will have documents giving an overview of the trial. You may make notes on the paper provided to take with you to the next station. In the next station you will be asked to speak with Mr. Smith. Please do not take the trial documents with you.

You have 1 minute reading time then a 9 minute prep station then a 10 minute communication station with an actor.

✏ Documents

The trial will compare a combination therapy to improve LUTS symptoms from BPH versus single agent therapy. The trial will be double-blinded and will involve adding a once-a-week medication to the patient's current medical therapy. The patient will either receive the active substance or a placebo. Suitable subjects will not have had previous surgical intervention on their prostate and will be on single therapy at the time of enrolment. They must undergo pre- and post- treatment urodynamics studies.

They will not have any major co-morbidities. Full information regarding the trial is available through the hospital's clinical trials lead and will be mailed or given to each subject. The trials unit has asked the urology team to approach potentially suitable patients and provide them with some information and, if they are interested, to pass their information to the trials coordinator who will contact them with further details and formally consent them.

COMMUNICATION

How would you begin?

Having introduced yourself, begin the consultation with an open question to assess the patient's understanding of the reason for the consultation.

You: "Hello my name is Dr. X, I am from the urology team. I have come to discuss the possibility of including you in a clinical trial. Can I start by asking what you have been told thus far?"

66 **Patient:** *"I have just seen the consultant who has said I could have a new tablet combination to help with my prostate problems."*

What would you ask next?

At this point you should continue to gather information on Mr. Smith's understanding of the treatment suggested. You should also consider an assessment of capacity to gauge Mr. Smith's ability to consent.

You: "Could you tell me what you understand the trial would involve?"

66   **Patient:** *"The doctor said it's a tablet that I take once a week for 6 months as well as the one I take at the minute."*

You: "That is correct."

What would you do next?

Having checked the patient's understanding of the trial at this stage it is sensible to assess the patient's concerns and expectations regarding the trial.

You: "What are you expecting from the trial? Do you have any particular worries?"

66   **Patient:** *"Well hopefully I am helping your boss with some research that could help others. I'm a bit worried that I might get some side-effects if it is a new drug to be honest."*

You: "I fully understand. Would you like me to explain a bit more in detail regarding how the trial works?"

66   **Patient:** *Yes please."*

Explain the trial to the patient

At this point, you will be required to deliver further information regarding the trial:

You: "This trial is a double blinded study. What this means is that neither you nor the researchers will know whether you are receiving the new drug, or a placebo. If you wished to participate in the study you would be asked to come to the hospital for urodynamics tests before starting the course of medication, and once again after the 6 months is up. These are tests that assess your bladder function and your urination. You would be followed up regularly both through phone calls from the research team and in person. You can pull out at any point and will be given information on who to contact at any time should you have any concern regarding potential side effects."

What would you do next?

At this point it would be prudent to check the patient's understanding. This will also allow you to clarify any important points.

You: "Is there anything that you would like me to go over again or any further questions you have?"

66   **Patient:** *"No that all makes sense doctor."*

How would you close the consultation?

The aim of your consultation is to gain consent from the patient if they decide to be part of the trial. If the patient is happy to participate in the trial then their information will be passed to the trials co-ordinator who will formally consent them.

You: "Thank you for your time Mr. Smith. To summarise we would like to include you in a double-blind trial that would involve adding in an extra tablet to your current medication regime and also having some urodynamic studies and seeing us in clinic at set intervals. Both the researchers and yourself would be unaware of which of the tablets you will be taking but both will be safe and if you were to develop any side-effects the tablet could be discontinued. You are free to leave the trial at any time. Are you happy for us to pass your information to the trials co-ordinator or would you like some time to think about it further?"

66 **Patient:** *"No, that sounds fine. I would be happy to be included in the trial and can fill in the paperwork. I just have a few questions if that is OK?"*

Please answer the patient's questions

66 *Patient: "What would happen if I wanted to stop taking the medication partly through the trial?"*

You: "You are within your rights to withdraw from the trial at any point. You do not have to provide a reason for this and this should not affect your subsequent treatment but you would be asked to let the tiral coordinators know about your decision."

66 **Patient:** *"Thanks. What would happen should I notice side effects from the new drug?"*

You: "You should report these to your local trial coordinator as soon as possible. Contact information will be provided with the information you receive should you decide to participate. These are considered as Serious Adverse Events (SAE) or Suspected Unexpected Serious Adverse Reactions (SUSAR) and need to be reported initially to the chief investigator and then to the sponsor."

SUMMARY

It is always good to start by assessing the level of the patient's knowledge prior to your consultation. Having done this you then can go on to inform them about the trial and fill in any gaps in their knowledge. It is important to address any patient concerns as you go along.

Whenever you are presented with a scenario that contains a signifianct amount of information, such as this station type with a designated 'prep station' it is vital that you effectively and succinctly pick out and summarise the salient points before you begin speaking with the patient/actor. For prep-stations you might wish to consider writing down the key points on scrap paper provided or simply highlighting key points. In this scenario there are a number of key points such as the double-blining and the need for pre- and post-treatment urodynamic studies.

Under the pressure of an OSCE it can be easy to forget certain aspects. The key is simply to remain calm in the prep-station, scan for the key information and then mentally summarise back to yourself the salient points. If you genuinely forget anything you can always be honest and simply say you will need to confirm with the trial co-ordinator or consultant and then get back to the patient.

COMMUNICATION

😐 **Actor Brief**

You are Peter Smith, a 76-year-old retired HGV driver. You are the main carer for your wife who suffers from dementia.

Presenting Complaint: You have longstanding problems with an enlarged prostate and the current medication has not improved your symptoms. You struggle to start passing urine, and often when you do the stream is poor. You wake several times throughout the night to pass urine and you have recently had several embarrassing "accidents" (post-voiding dribbling) when people have come to visit.

ICE: You are not keen for surgery as do not want to have periods of time away from your wife and therefore are keen to try other medication.

Significant PMH/DH/SH: Non-smoker, with high blood pressure.

TOP TIPS

➕ Ensure use of layman's terms throughout when discussing the intricacies of the trial.

➕ Regular checking of understanding is essential when you are imparting large volumes of information such as in this case.

➕ The final decision is the patient's and if they do not wish to enter the trial you should respect their decision.

2.9 | Consent: Cholecystectomy

Scenario

You are the SHO in clinic with Mr. Johnson, consultant hepatopancreatobiliary surgeon. As this is a busy clinic your consultant has asked if you wouldn't mind helping speed up the process by utilising a spare consultation room and consenting Mrs. Kimberley Hemsworth, who is a 37-year-old overweight lady who is suffering from biliary colic and requires a laparoscopic cholecystectomy. Please explain the procedure and get the patient to sign a consent form.

How would you begin?

Begin with an introduction of yourself and the role you are playing within today's' consultation and confirming what she knows about the condition and procedure. You have already confirmed you have the correct patient.

You: "Hello, my name is Dr. X and I'm one of the doctors on Mr. Johnson's surgical team. He has asked me to run through the consent process for this procedure but first I would like to confirm what you know about your condition and what you know about the procedure itself?"

❝ **Patient:** "I know that I have some stones in my gall bladder but to be honest I don't really care, I just want this thing out and to be back to my normal self."

Please consent the patient

Use signposting to explain what is required. This will help provide structure and focus the scenario on getting the form signed within the allocated time.

You: "OK, shall we run through this consent form and please feel free to ask any questions along the way. I'll explain about what has been happening in your body, the treatment options, the potential issues and what will happen on the day. "

❝ **Patient:** "OK, that sounds fine."

You: "Gallstones are formed when there is an imbalance of certain chemicals in the gall bladder. Although many of the population can live with gallstones and never be aware of them, some people do develop symptoms and problems associated with gallstones. The most serious complication being pancreatitis, an inflammation of the pancreas gland, which can make you quite unwell. "

❝ **Patient:** "Are there any alternatives to surgery?"

You: "In terms of alternative treatment, there is little to offer you. Although a significant number of the population carry gallstones, you have already had symptoms and would be at risk of further attacks. If you would not like to proceed with surgery, we can keep you as a patient in this clinic here, seeing you periodically, or we can discharge you with a view to being seen at your request."

🖊 Comm Skills Tip: Alternatives To Surgery

As per consenting guidelines, you should offer alternative treatment options. What alternatives are there for the treatment of biliary colic?

The initial management of biliary colic is analgesia, surgery should be considered if recurrent symptoms do not respond to analgesia. It must be noted that the coexistence of pain and the presence of gallstones does not guarantee causation, as demonstrated by those patients who continue to experience the pain that had been attributed to billiary colic despite cholecytectomy.

Realistically there are few alternatives other than surgical for the management of biliary colic. Traditionally a low fat diet was advised on the basis that fat in the diet stimulates cholecytokinin mediated gall bladder contraction but studies have not found this to be effective in reducing symptoms.

❝ Patient: "I'm a little worried about having an operation. What are the risks?"

There are a lot of complications that the patient must be aware to allow informed consent:
• Bleeding (right hepatic artery, cystic artery bud)
• Infection (LRTI, pneumonia, wound, urine, intra-abdominal)
• Conversion to open procedure
• Damage to common hepatic / bile duct requiring further operation to repair (<1%)
• Perforation of viscus
• Scars
• Anaesthetic risk

You: "There are some risks with this operation that I need to make you aware of. As we'll be making a cut there is a risk of scarring and bleeding, both internally and at the skin. There is a risk of infection, of the wound itself and on the inside as well in the lungs and the bladder. Overall less than 5% of patients undergoing this procedure would need to be converted to an open operation, meaning that instead of several small cuts, there would be a large cut. An open operation usually means a longer hospital stay and recovery. Due to the nature of the relations of the gall bladder there is a small risk of damaging some of the structures around it, which we would try to deal with at the time of the operation. As the procedure will involve you being asleep, there is a small risk of a reaction to the anaesthetic, you will be able to discuss any questions regarding the anaesthetic with your anaesthetist on the day of the procedure."

❝ Patient: "When my sister had a bowel operation she needed a blood transfusion afterwards. Might I need something like that?"

Are there any additional procedures you should consent Miss Hemsworth for?

Although not a particular risk in this lady, there is a small chance that she might need an on table cholangiogram. If she bleeds a lot there is also a small chance of requiring a blood transfusion. A bile leak may require a drain to be inserted.

You: "Additional procedures are uncommon during this procedure, though there is a small chance we'd need to do some x-rays, perform a blood transfusion and you may require a surgical drain."

Patient: "Who will actually be doing the operation? Will it be Mr. Johnson the consultant?"

How would you respond?

Although the surgery would be officially performed under a named consultant, Mr. Johnson in this example, the patient should be aware that it may not be Mr. Johnson specifically performing the operation. A member of the team, who is adequately qualified, could be the person to perform the procedure.

You: "Unfortunately, I cannot make promises on behalf of Mr. Johnson. Either Mr. Johnson, or a suitably qualified member of his team will perform the operation on the day. "

Patient: "Well I'm quite anxious about things now."

Now would be a good time to show empathy for the patient's anxiety and also to explore her ideas, concerns and expectations and help to reassure her.

You: " I fully understand. Having an operation can be a scary experience and it is my job to explain all the potential risks to you today, which can make things, sound much worse. Is there anything about the operation that is particularly worrying you?"

Patient: "Well I have a dog to look after. Can this be done as a day case?"

There are specific guidelines that should be followed when considering whether a patient is appropriate to be considered for a day case list. There are exclusion lists and inclusion lists. Exclusion criteria can include a high BMI, MI within 6 months, uncontrollable hypertension, heart failure and ASA >2.

You: "Patient safety is our highest priority and although we would like to make this as easy as possible for you, I believe in your particular case it would be safer to do this as an inpatient."

Patient: "OK, but will I be able to live normally without my gallbladder?"

The gallbladder is not an essential organ for life and there are few sequelae following successful removal.

You: "The gall bladder is a small sac that is placed under the liver and it's function is to store and squirt out bile when you eat. The body can comfortable live without the gallbladder without any real long term problems."

Patient: "OK, thanks I feel much more confident about the operation now and I would like to sign the consent form."

COMMUNICATION

SUMMARY

Consenting a patient is an incredibly important surgical process. Patient expectation must be managed appropriately so there are no surprises and unnecessary anxiety and, potentially, medico-legal issues can be avoided. The risks of laparoscopic cholecystectomy are generally low in the absence of inflammation (< 5% conversion, < 0.5% bile duct injury) but the risks increase with established cholecystitis or acute pancreatitis.

Gallstones are often the result of inequality between three delicately balanced components – phospholipids, lecithin and bile salts (Admirand's triangle). This causes a build up of one component forming one of three different stones – cholesterol, bilirubin or mixed. Potential complications include – biliary colic, cholecystitis, choledocholithiasis, ascending cholangitis, biliary perforation, mucocoele, pancreatitis and gall stone ileus.

(☺) **Actor brief**

You are Kimberley Hemsworth, a 37 year married lady with 3 children. You work at the local supermarket and are known by many in your local village as being the life and soul of the party. You love your family and live for friendly interaction with other people. You like life's little things, though this you are a self-confessed lover of food and alcohol and know you should probably lose weight, which you put on after having your children but never got around to actively getting fit.

Presenting Complaint: You initially had some pain in your right upper quadrant over a year ago now which was the worst pain you'd ever experienced. You ended up going to the emergency department via an ambulance and was given a lot of morphine to calm the pain down. Although you only spent one night on the surgical ward it was one of the worst experiences of life in terms of pain. You were discharged following a resolution of the pain, normal blood results and an ultrasound scan which confirmed the presence of gallstones. Sadly, you missed your outpatient appointment and had 3 further attacks of colic after this. You are now desperate to have this operation.

ICE: You're not really sure about what is involved with the operation but you are sure you don't want a big scar as you're already not particularly proud of body as it is. You expect that the operation will go smoothly as you aren't really aware of anything that could go wrong.

TOP TIPS

➕ Pay attention to the brief. If it states that you must get the actor to sign the consent form as part of the station make sure that you do so.

➕ Signposting is a great way to manage time and also guide the actor through the steps of the consultation.

2.10 | Consent: Dynamic Hip Screw

Scenario

You are the Trauma and Orthopaedics SHO on-call being shadowed by a medical student. You have seen a pleasant 80-year-old lady, who lives in her own home, in the emergency department having been brought in by an ambulance. She has fallen over in the lounge and landed on her left-hand side with immediate pain and deformity of the left leg. You suspect a hip fracture, which is confirmed as an inter-trochanteric fracture by a pelvic x-ray. Your registrar is currently unavailable as he is in emergency theatre with a poly-trauma patient. As you have seen and clerked the patient, you have decided to take it upon yourself to consent the patient for the procedure, which you believe would be a dynamic hip screw.

How would you begin?

Begin with an introduction of your accompanying medical student and yourself, the role you are playing in today's' consultation and confirming what she knows about the condition and procedure. You have already confirmed you have the correct patient.

You: "Hello, my name is Dr. X and I'm one of the doctors on the Trauma and Orthopaedic surgical team and this is Matthew, one of our medical students who is observing if that is OK? Can I ask you to confirm exactly what you understand has happened?"

❝ Patient: "Well, a young man kindly came along and told me that I'd broken my hip and that it wouldn't fix itself but would need fixing with an operation. Is that right?"

How would you explain the operation to the patient?

You: "I have been asked to explain to you a bit more about the operation and to get you to sign this consent form if you are happy to proceed with the operation. Is that OK?"

❝ Patient: "Yes thank you."

You: "OK, shall we run through this consent form and please feel free to ask any questions along the way. I'll explain about what has been happening with your hip, the treatment options, the potential issues and what will happen on the day. "

❝ Patient: "OK."

Explain what is the nature of her injury and what will happen without operative intervention? What are the benefits of surgery?

Hip fractures are common yet are a surgical emergency requiring operative intervention to treat most effectively. The risks can drastically affect the patients' potential quality of life.

You: "As you correctly said you have broken your hip. While this is a common injury it is quite a big injury. The operation we will perform will involve us fixing the fracture with a screw and plate known as a dynamic hip screw. The beauty of the operation is that you will be able to walk on your hip the next day after the operation. Before the operation was

COMMUNICATION

used patients would need to stay in bed on traction for 8 weeks for the fracture to heal and this led to lots of complications."

What are the risks of surgery that you would consent the patient for?

The risks of having a hip fracture fixed are varied and include:
• Bleeding – wound, intra-operative
• Infection – wound, chest, urine
• Malunion, non-union
• Sciatic nerve injury
• Numbness
• DVT / PE
• Anaesthetic risk

You: "Although it is a good operation it is not without risk. You will have a long cut on the outside of your hip when you wake up which will have clips or stitches. Occasionally this can leak and there is a chance that you might pick up an infection in the wound, your chest or urine while you are less mobile than normal. As you will be less mobile there is also an increased risk of picking up a blood clot in the legs or lungs, we will give you some blood thinning injections to reduce the risk of this but it can still occur. As we cut through the skin there is a risk of damaging nerves near the skin and you might notice that the area around the scar feels numb. From a technical point of view there is a small chance that the screw and plate might fail or the bone not heal correctly, if this were to happen you might require a further operation."

What are the alternatives to surgery for this patient?

As a broad rule almost all patients with hip fractures will be managed surgically in some form or another. Those who are for non-operative management are generally very poor candidates for theatre, including those who are moribund or those with significant co-morbidities. Without treatment the patient could not be realistically expected to ever have a reasonable level of functional mobility and would need to stay bed-bound for eight weeks.

You: "In terms of the fracture, these generally do quite poorly when left to heal by themselves, often taking months to do so with poor results, and so generally it is recommended that these types of fracture are fixed with an operation. For your particular fracture we would use what is called a dynamic hip screw, a type of metal bolt that secures the fracture in place and allows it to heal while you walk on it."

Are there any additional procedures you would consent Mrs. Jones for?

You: "During the procedure you might lose some blood and require a blood transfusion following surgery."

Patient: "OK, as long as it's put right. I'm concerned about going under a general anaesthetic though as I've been feeling more and more frail. I'm not sure that my body could take this?"

You: "Your concern for general anaesthetic is understandable, though for the vast majority of patients it is a very safe and acceptable method of operating. A common alternative is a spinal anaesthetic, which puts less strain on your heart and lungs. The anaesthetist will come and see you closer to the time of the operation and will be more than happy to discuss your concerns."

COMMUNICATION

66 **Patient:** "Well, I don't want to feel any pain. What will happen after the operation? Will I be able to walk?"

The post-operative period following hip fracture fixation is of the utmost importance. It is important to manage her expectations of the operation and her recovery. Although a hip fracture is a major insult to the body, with some sources quoting a 30% mortality within a year from the fracture itself and associated issues, there is also a high expectation of the patient to be able to mobilise with physiotherapy on the first day after the operation.

You: "As mentioned you will be able to walk straight away. Due to the nature of the injury and the operation the hip will be quite sore and you will likely need a frame or sticks to walk with the aid of the physios. It can take a good few months (up to 6-12 in some cases) to regain both your confidence and full mobility. The stitches or clips will be taken out in around 2 weeks once the wound has healed."

66 **Patient:** "Gosh that seems fast, I'm not sure I'll be able to manage that but I'll give it a try!"

How will you close the consultation?

To finish a consultation, it is always important to briefly summarise what has been discussed and what the forward management plan. Not only does this improve communication between doctor and patient but also, in the exam setting, can enable you to demonstrate your own understanding of the situation.

You: "OK Mrs. Jones, I would just like to summarise some of the information we have shared today. You have broken your hip, which will require an operation to fix, there are some risks, which we have been through today, but there also significant benefits, including getting you back on your feet from the day after the operation. If you are happy I would like you to sign here on the consent form."

66 **Patient:** "Yes, thank you that will be fine."

COMMUNICATION

SUMMARY

Extracapsular hip fractures and subsequent dynamic hip screw fixation and consent is extremely common. The main risks to the patient are those of immobility such as thrombosis and infection rather than less frequent technical risks like failure of the metalwork or malunion and nonunion of the bone.

The key aspects to DHS consent are emphasising that although there is the option for non-operative management this is really only reserved for those who will almost certainly not survive an operation since the purpose of intervening surgically is to get the patient walking as soon as possible to reduce the high morbidity and mortality statistics (30% at 30 days and 30% at a year respectively).

Given the impact the injury will have on the patient's mobility it is also vital to outline the post-operative recovery and to appropriately manage the patient's expectations.

🙂 **Actor Brief**

You are Mrs. Grace Jones, an 80-year-old daughter of a Welsh miner and house-wife. You recently moved into a residential home as your daughter had been concerned for your welfare, she had said that you were becoming increasingly and intermittently forgetful and repeating yourself too often. You don't really see what the trouble has been about, though your GP also seems concerned as he's started you on some "memory tablets". Recently you have noticed that you're starting to struggle with your mobility and have stopped going outside.

Presenting Complaint Whilst walking through the communal area in the residential home you tripped over a pouf placed inconveniently.

ICE You're not really sure about what is involved with the operation but you are sure you don't want a big scar as you're already not particularly proud of body as it is. You expect that the operation will go smoothly as you aren't really aware of anything that could go wrong.

PMH
Hypercholesterolaemia
Osteoporosis
IHD
COPD

COMMUNICATION

TOP TIPS

➕ There is a lot of information to cover and it can be easy to over-load the actor/patient with information. Give the risks in bite-size chunks such as those related to immobility *(thrombosis and infec-tion)*, those related to the wound *(ooze)* and technical aspects such as failure and malunion and nonunion.

➕ Try to avoid using too many technical terms. While it is good that you know the anatomy around the hip joint it is not always neces-sary to inform the patient of this and it can inhibit their overall understanding of what needs to happen.

2.11 | Consent: Flexible Sigmoidoscopy

Scenario

You are the SHO in Mr. Khan's busy colorectal clinic seeing Mr. Sterling, a 32-year-old businessman who has been troubled with abdominal pain and PR bleeding. Mr. Khan has already seen the patient and is wondering whether the patient has proctitis, possibly due to inflammatory bowel disease. He would like a flexible sigmoidoscopy performing when the patient has had adequate bowel preparation in the next few days.

You have washed your hands, introduced yourself and confirmed you have the correct patient. Please take Mr. Sterling through the consenting process for this procedure.

How would you begin?

Open questions are always a great way to begin a consultation. Start with checking Mr. Sterling's understanding about what is happening and what the proposed management plan is.

You: "Could I begin by briefly asking just exactly what has happened and what you understand by what Mr. Khan has said about how we move forward?"

❝ **Patient:** "Yes, of course, I have been experiencing some strange abdominal pain and passing large amounts of blood from the back passage. I've asked Mr. Khan what he believed it may be and he suggested that it could be what my mum and dad have or something else, like a polyp I think he said. He mentioned a "sigi", though I'm not entirely sure what that means?"

How would you explain the nature of the differential diagnosis?

It would be difficult to only have one differential diagnosis at this point, though his symptoms seem to be describing more of a proctitis than anything else. Potential differentials for a gentleman in this age group could include an anal fissure, haemorrhoids, IBD, rectal polyp or colorectal carcinoma.

You: "Mr. Khan believes that there may be something going on, which could include the same issues your mother and father have or it could be something else. The best way forward would be to physically look at the bowel lining itself and possibly take a biopsy at the same time."

Mr. Sterling is clearly unaware of the what a flexible sigmoidoscopy is as Mr. Khan appears to have used a colloquialism. How would you describe this procedure to Mr. Sterling?

You: "Mr. Khan was referring to a procedure called a flexible sigmoidoscopy, which is essentially a fine camera that is passed into the back passage to have a look at the lining of the bowel directly. It can be very useful in helping diagnose or exclude conditions that could be responsible for the complaints that you have had. The procedure itself lasts between 10-20 minutes and is generally very well tolerated by patients."

COMMUNICATION

66 **Patient:** "Gosh, I don't like the idea of having something shoved up my back passage! Are there any alternatives?"

There are increasingly viable alternative options that can be sought if flexible sigmoidoscopy is not an attractive option. Full colonoscopy would be able to visualize the entirety of the colon. If endoscopy cannot be pursued, a CT abdomen could be performed but with ever increasing resolutions of CT scanners, a more specific "CT Colon" could be performed, though this would not allow histological investigation.

You: "Endoscopy would be the investigation of choice as it would allow us to physically see the lining of your bowel, though if this is an unacceptable option for you then there are alternatives such as having a CT scan of your abdomen though the reliability at spotting a diagnosis is not as good."

66 **Patient:** "I've heard these CT scans can give you cancer from the radiation. I think I'd rather we went ahead with the flexible sigmoidoscopy, can you tell me anything more about it? What are its benefits?"

Sigmoidoscopy can be both diagnostic and therapeutic. As mentioned the major benefit of having flexible sigmoidoscopy is that there can be a direct visualization of the bowel mucosa In addition to this the endoscopist can take a biopsy or perform polypectomy.

You: "At the time of the procedure, the endoscopist can directly inspect the inner lining of your bowel, which can help to narrow down the diagnosis. They can also take a sample of your tissue and send it to a specialized doctor who will look down a microscope to examine it and provide us with further details. If polyps are found there may be an opportunity to cut them out meaning that part of the problem will have been dealt with."

66 **Patient:** "That sounds great."

What are the risks of this procedure?

There are risks associated with endoscopy including bowel perforation, sedative reaction, bleeding and failure of procedure.

You: "Unfortunately, there are risks with any procedure. With this procedure it is possible but rare to have some bleeding and discomfort at the time of the operation as well as afterwards. There is also a small risk that hole can be made in the bowel lining, which could represent a serious problem, potentially requiring an operation to fix. There is also a small chance that you can react to the sedative."

Patient: "OK, I accept there's always a risk with anything, just as long as I get someone who knows what they're doing! What kind of anaesthetic will I get?"

Most patients are able to tolerate the procedure without ill effect or sedation, though some patients may find parts of the procedure uncomfortable and be offered sedation in the form of a benzodiazepine. In reality, it would be difficult to discuss this with the patient fully as you would not be performing the procedure yourself.

You: "Many patients are quite comfortable during the procedure, though if you have any concerns you can discuss these beforehand with your endoscopist."

What would you warn the patient about after the procedure?

Bowel perforation is a serious but rare risk of the procedure and the patient should have safety netting as to the signs and symptoms of this condition as well as what to do in this event.

You: "Although rare, occasionally there is a hole in the bowel made by the procedure, if this does happen you may experience a disproportionate amount of abdominal pain and find your stomach goes rigid, if this is the case you must present to the emergency department for immediate medical assessment."

66 **Patient:** "OK, I understand."

What else does this patient need to know in terms of pre-operative preparation?

In order to properly visualise the bowel mucosa the patient will require bowel prep. This is in the form of clear liquids only for 12 hours before hand as well as a laxative the night before and an enema.

You: "Preparation for the procedure actually begins the night before in the form of only drinking clear fluids for 12 hours prior to your allocated time and having both a laxative and a sedative."

How would you finish the consultation?

Finishing a consultation can be very important in terms of confirming the information that has been exchanged and managing expectations.

You: "OK Mr. Sterling, let's just re-cap so if there's anything wrong we can correct it now. We would like to perform a flexible sigmoidoscopy, which will allow us to see the bowel and take some samples, with a view to narrowing down the cause of your symptoms. There are some risks with the procedure, which we have gone over. We would need you to prepare the night before by adhering to our specific regime to help clear out the bowel. We will see you again in the clinic with the results and forward action plan."

SUMMARY

Flexible sigmoidoscopy offers a minimally invasive technique to allow visualisation of the large bowel up to 60cm from the anus. In conditions of the sigmoid colon and rectum it can provide a relatively quick and sage technique to allow diagnosis.

Although performed only under sedation it is usually well-tolerated though this can put some patients off. When consenting it is important to explain that bowel preparation will be required in order to allow for proper visualisation by the endoscopist.

COMMUNICATION

😐 Actor Brief

You are Mark Sterling, a 32 year old business man desperately trying to climb the corporate ladder in a management and sales team in a busy textile factory. You have always aspired to be as rich as possible, not necessarily through greed but rather as you see yourself as the main breadwinner for your young family and you want the best for them. You have 3 children at home, all young and requiring their mother, your wife Chloe, to have given up her job to take care of them. You take your lifestyle and your health very seriously and are very pleased you have got to see a doctor about this problem. You enjoy racket sports, especially squash and badminton and enjoy taking your children to see the great outdoors.

Presenting Complaint For the past 3 months you have been experiencing more and more fresh red blood in the pan. Although the amount of blood scares you, the defaecation process is actually relieving, as the pain tends to go away when you have finished. You have recently noticed your right thumb aching though you put this down to the hefty amount of squash you have been playing.

ICE You are unsure as to the cause of this problem, though you are concerned that it might be cancer, as you saw some posters in your GP surgery warning you about this.

PMH Nil

SH Non-smoker, occasional alcohol, international sales manager (Africa East) for a textiles company

DH Nil regular, NKDA

FH Father – Crohn's disease; Mother – Ulcerative colitis

TOP TIPS

➕ Don't assume that just because a patient has seen a consultant that they understand everything about the operation. It may be that they can't recall the discussion or forgot to ask some important questions at the intial consultation.

➕ Don't forget to include biopsy and polypectomy to the consent form as endoscopy can also be interventional.

2.12 Angry Relative: Wrong Diagnosis

Scenario

It is 8:30pm. You are the orthopaedic SHO just starting a night shift. You are on the paediatric ward to explain to an angry mother that her daughter Jessica (9 years old) does not need an MUA of her fractured left wrist and can go home tonight. The ED doctor had already told them an operation was needed. You and your consultant Ms. Tarker have already seen the x-ray and heard the history/examination findings from ED. Ms. Tarker wants the patient managed in a backslab with follow up in fracture clinic in one week's time. (The fracture is a left distal radial buckle fracture with minimal angulation/loss of radial height and no neurovascular deficit and ED have already applied an appropriate backslab).

Please take a brief history and explain to the mother of the patient that an MUA is not indicated. Then explain the conservative management plan and that they can go home.

How would you begin?

You: "Good evening, is it Mrs. Bilker and Jessica?"

66 **Mother:** "Yes. Who are you?"

You: "My name is Dr. X, I'm the night doctor for Trauma and Orthopaedics. I'm sorry my daytime colleague did not get a chance to see you, unfortunately there is only one doctor on for day/night shifts that deals with emergency admissions and it was a very busy day." (An early apology can help. The patient/relative may still want to vent their grievances but it sets the tone for the conversation.)

66 **Mother:** "Yes well we've been waiting over 5 hours now! Neither of us has eaten since lunchtime and we've been told nothing in ages. Jessica needs an operation!"

You: "I'm sorry you've had a long day and that you haven't been kept informed, let me see if we can work towards correcting that now. I understand the Emergency doctor told you Jessica needs an operation. Please can you just tell me how she injured herself again so that I have the full story?"

66 **Mother:** "Like I already told them in A&E, she was skateboarding about 3pm and fell on her left hand. And before you ask, no she didn't hit her head, no she doesn't have any allergies and yes she's otherwise completely healthy. When is she having her operation?!" (Jessica corroborates this story, there is good rapport with her mother and no features suggesting a NAI)

How will you respond?

You: "I can see you've already been through this all before. What exactly did the Emergency doctor tell you?"

> **Mother:** "He said she'd broken her left wrist and that it was kind of bent. That it needed straightening out with an operation – a manipulation or something."

What will you ask next?

Now is a good opportunity to assess the mother's ideas, concerns and expectations.
You: "And is there anything in particular you're worried about?"

> **Mother:** "Well OBVIOUSLY I don't want her to have a wonky arm!!! How long does this operation take?" [becoming more angry]

You: "I can understand why that might worry you. I know you've been told that Jessica needs an operation but in actual fact she doesn't and I would like to go through this with you now to explain why and to answer any questions you might have."

> **Mother:** "WHAT?!?! No operation?!! You're kidding!"

You: "Mrs. Bilker (and Jessica), the type of break that Jessica has sustained is what we call a buckle fracture – the bone is not snapped cleanly in two, instead it has been squashed slightly. Now in adults this wouldn't happen but in children the bone is still a bit soft. Children are also much better at healing and remodelling their bones. What this means is that although there is a buckle fracture of Jessica's wrist, she will heal well and overtime the bone will remodel and straighten out so that you'd never know it was broken in the first place."

> **Mother:** "Won't an operation be better to get it straight. Are you sure you're not just trying to save money for the NHS. I don't want my daughter to have a deformed arm!"

You: "I understand your worries completely, this is absolutely nothing to do with saving money. This is about doing what's best for Jessica. In fact I've already discussed Jessica's x-ray with the consultant, Ms. Tarker, and she has advised that an operation is not appropriate. I know you were told an operation was needed and I'm sorry that this was inaccurate but Ms. Tarker is more senior than the doctor you saw in the emergency department and she is the orthopaedic consultant (bone specialist) on call today which is why our team's opinion was sought. Ms. Tarker has advised that an operation isn't needed and would likely make Jessica worse off. This is a very common injury that we manage in a cast/backslab but we would follow Jessica up in our fracture clinic to make sure everything is healing as planned. Like I explained there will likely be no significant sign of the injury in time. Her bone will remodel and heal up."

> **Mother:** "Wow. I wish someone had explained this sooner. We're tired, starving and frankly fed up."

How would you close the consultation?

You: "Mrs. Bilker, I sympathise completely. Just so I haven't missed anything let me recap everything and if you have any remaining questions we can address those too. Jessica fell this afternoon and suffered a buckle fracture of her left wrist. She is otherwise fit and well and did not suffer any other injuries other than some grazing to her palm and knee. The x-ray has been reviewed by myself and the consultant and the best way to manage this injury is with a backslab and simple painkillers initially. There is no need for surgery, which would not add any benefit and could likely do more harm. The good news is that Jessica has the backslab already on. We will book you into our fracture clinic in a week's time to see how Jessica is getting on and there's no reason why you both can't go home now. So Jessica can definitely have something to eat - we can arrange the ward to provide something now if you don't want to wait until you get home. Do you have any other questions?" (Remembering that the patient is hungry is a nice touch – it shows you've fully listened, not just to the medical aspects.)

66 **Mother:** "No thank you for explaining everything. It's been a long day but I'm grateful you've cleared everything up, thank you."

SUMMARY

Forearm fractures in children are common making up about 40% of childhood fractures. They are often managed conservatively. Children heal more quickly than adults. As a rough guide where an adult fracture takes on average 6 weeks to heal, many paediatric fractures heal in 3-4 weeks. This trends towards 6 weeks as they reach skeletal maturity. The principles of fracture management can still be simply thought of as: reduce, immobilise, analgesia (never forget pain relief!) and rehabilitate.
Other factors affecting bone healing are: smoking, diabetes, immunosuppression, anatomy (non-union is common in the scaphoid, navicular and talus), type of fracture (open vs closed, simple vs comminuted, soft tissue damage, ie forces from mechanism of injury). Pick a way to categorise these aspects for the exam: local, systemic, congenital for example.

😐 Actor Brief

You are Mrs. Bilker, mother of Jessica, an 9 year old girl who fell onto concrete with her left hand outstretched while out skateboarding this afternoon around 3pm.

You have sat in ED for 5 hours and have just been transferred up to the paediatric ward without being seen yet by the T+O doctor. The ED doctor (F2) has said that the x-ray shows a break in the left wrist and that this will need an operation to put it into a better position. (MUA). You have not been told anything else. Jessica has been kept NBM and last ate at 12pm. You are furious about lack of communication, waiting to be seen and Jessica is upset about not being allowed to eat.

Presenting Complaint: Jessica was out skateboarding with friends on the street outside your house at 3pm. She fell over on an outstretched left hand and sustained grazing to her left palm and left knee. She did not hit her head/lose consciousness. She ran inside crying and that's when she noticed her wrist was also very sore.

ICE: You are very concerned about Jessica having a deformed arm/impaired function. You've been told she needs an operation. You wonder if the change in plan is to do with saving money and suspect the doctor is trying to cut corners by not operating (which is not the case).

COMMUNICATION

You are also furious about: waiting, lack of clear communication – being shipped up to ward without knowing what is going to happen next and are even more angry when you are told you can go home and that no operation is needed.

PMH/DH/SH: Jessica is fit and well, non-smoking household, right hand dominant, lives with mother/father and younger brother (7yo).

Special Instructions: You are very angry (see ICE section for details). The doctor needs to utter the words 'I'm sorry' in an appropriate context for you to start settling down. Only appropriate explanation (ie that surgery would not make this better and could make it worse and is definitely not indicated in this type of injury) allows you to calm down enough to agree to go home. You also need significant reassurance that everything appropriate has and will be done (backslab, follow up plan etc) and that Jessica is highly unlikely to suffer any lasting disability.

TOP TIPS

➕ There is no way around it, you must apologise in order to make progress with this communication skills station, she is understandably angry and worried. In order to make positive steps towards getting her to agree to go home you will need to address this first. Specific things that can be apologised for are: the long wait in ED, not seeing the T+O day doctor, the misinformation from the ED doctor – the key thing here would be to say that while they thought an operation was needed you have since consulted with someone much senior/more experienced/a bone expert who has seen the x-ray and advised that surgery is not the right thing to do for Jessica

➕ Once the apology is given, move towards educating the mother, reassuring her and explaining that Jessica will be closely followed up. Then broach the subject of going home. Addressing the mother's ICE will be key.

➕ If there is a mother and child in the scenario *(rather than just the mother)* make sure you confirm the identity of the adult with the patient *(in this case it's her mother)* and also include Jessica in your discussion/ask if she has any questions.

➕ Make sure you're satisfied with the history/timeline. ALWAYS consider non-accidental injury in any child you see.

2.13 | Angry Patient: Self-Discharge

Scenario

You are the on-call SHO on a general surgical ward at night; the nurses have bleeped you to see a patient, Mr. Markham, you assessed earlier who has been waiting for a registrar review. Clinically his situation remains unchanged and is most likely appendicitis. The patient has become agitated about the long waiting time, as the registrar is tied up with a difficult Hartmann's procedure in theatre, and now wants to leave. You have washed your hands and introduced yourself. Please take a history and suggest a management plan.

How would you begin?

You: "Hello Mr. Markham, I'm very sorry about the wait. My Name is Dr. X from the surgical team. I understand that you are unable to stay in the hospital for assessment?"

❝ Patient: "Listen, I'm not being funny but I've been waiting in this hospital for 6 hours now and I'm still no closer to knowing why I feel so unwell! I have a job and responsibilities; I can't afford to be off work! Just exactly when am I going to be seen by someone who actually knows what they're doing?!"

What would you ask next?

As the patient is angry he will likely not have registered your apology. A second apology and open question asked in a calm manner will help build rapport. Body language is key, try not to look aggressive or threatening, turn your body diagonally so as not to appear to be "squaring up" and actively listen to his concerns.

You: "I can see you're quite upset at the moment and I apologise again for the delay, is there anything else worrying you?"

❝ Patient: "I've been waiting in this hospital for hours now. All I want to know is what is causing me to feel this way?! You said your registrar will come down and have a chat with me but when is this going to happen? I have a young daughter I need to look after!"

What would you ask next?

This is now the best time to ask about the patient's ideas, concerns and expectations. Apologising for the situation does not convey guilt nor blame and should be encouraged to help with the process. Offer the patient information that makes them aware that the registrar is still busy with an emergency but that they will be reviewed as soon as possible.

You: "I'm very sorry you have experienced this, unfortunately the registrar is stuck with an emergency at this time, though he is aware of you and your situation. What do you think is the cause of your pain? I understand you are concerned for your daughter, have you got any other concerns at all?"

❝ Patient: "I don't know what is happening with my stomach but it is starting to concern me. I didn't have the chance to organise anyone to pick up my daughter from school with all this going on and I'm worried she'll be alone when school finishes.

COMMUNICATION

My brother lives nearby and could look after her but I've been unable to contact him as I don't get phone reception in this hospital."

The patient has presented you with an issue that can be solved with a simple phone call using one of the hospital phones. The specific example is almost unimportant, more that there is a problem to be solved that could convince the patient to stay and win back his trust.

You: "If we can provide you with a phone, would you be convinced to stay?"

66 **Patient:** "That would be very helpful, thank you, though I feel we're not achieving anything if I do stay as this hospital seems to be very inefficient."

What else would you like to ask?

It seems that you are at the end of the road in terms of problems that you can help with. Now is the time to check the patient's understanding of the current clinical situation and to express your concerns about his welfare.

You: "Earlier I felt as though the cause of your abdominal pain could be appendicitis, what do you understand by this?"

66 **Patient:** "Well, I've had a look on google and it says it's a problem with the appendix that needs an operation to take it away, otherwise it can be quite dangerous but I really do need to go."

The patient has already researched the problem and clearly has capacity with a statement like this. He is still choosing to leave the hospital and you cannot stop him from doing so. You can still present your professional opinion to him and inform him of the natural course of appendicitis without surgical intervention.

You: "I see that you've researched what we think it may be. Although the diagnosis as of yet is unclear, if you do feel like you have to leave we can still offer you some treatment in the form of antibiotics. Even though you're leaving the hospital that does not mean that we can't look after you in the future, this hospital is a 24-hour service and we'd be more than happy to see you again should this issue not resolve or even get worse. "

66 **Patient:** "That's great, thank you."

What must be done prior to this patient leaving hospital medico-legally? What is included on this form?

The patient must sign a form to state that he is leaving contrary to medical advice. The form should clearly state the name of the patient and the potential diagnosis. It should include any safety-netting that is necessary and that the patient understands the risk they are taking upon themselves.

Before leaving the patient has a few questions for you

66 **Patient:** "What kind of things do I need to look out for to tell me its getting worse?"

You: "I would recommend returning as soon as possible if you notice worsening pain, your tummy becomes tense or rigid or if you develop a worsening fever or vomiting symptoms."

66 **Patient:** "OK, thanks I'll do that but I really have to go."

SUMMARY

Appendicitis is one of the most common general surgical emergency presentations. In England approximately 50 000 appendicectomies are performed each year. The aetiology of appendicitis is often not clear. Proposed causes include intra-luminal blockage (stool, foreign body, parasites), blockage secondary to appendiceal wall swelling (lymphoid hyperplasia, tumour) inflammatory bowel disease and trauma.

The classical natural history of appendicitis is for the blockage to cause luminal venous thrombosis, followed by engorgement, anti-mesenteric ischaemia, perforation which can lead to abscess formation, peritonitis and death. It has been proposed that the condition may also spontaneously resolve itself and some episodes may even be sub-clinical although this is not universally acknowledged.

Dealing with angry patients is almost universally made easier by first acknowledging their displeasure and asking open questions to allow them to explain what has happened. Apologising on behalf of the hospital for their situation not only acknowledges the patient's anguish but also shows you care about the patient.
When a patient has capacity you cannot stop them from making their own autonomous decisions. You can, however, provide them with your medical opinion and recommendations. Safety netting in this case is of paramount importance, not only for your own peace of mind in providing the best possible care but also in terms of patient safety and medico-legal responsibility for the hospital. In this case offering the patient solutions to current problems (phone call to brother), providing immediate (antibiotics TTO) and future (coming back to the hospital) treatment should satisfy yourself that you have done the utmost for this patient.

COMMUNICATION

😐 Actor Brief

You are Christopher Markham, a 28 year old ex-IVDU who fell in with the wrong crowd when you were younger, developing a minor criminal record and acquiring status as a single father of a 5 year old daughter, of whom you are completely dedicated to. You have now been discharged from counselling and rehab, with your life getting back on track with a steady, if somewhat poorly paid, factory worker job. You haven't touched drugs or alcohol for some time now but do make occasional poor choices. Your 5 year old daughter, Millie, is actually home alone as a co-worker at the factory phoned for an ambulance and you haven't had the chance to make alternative care arrangements.

Presenting Complaint: Your abdominal pain actually started the night before but as you're desperate for the money from your job you ignored the pain as much as possible. The pain itself seems to have changed and appears to be migrating. You have been unable to eat today as you have simply felt too nauseous and sweaty.

ICE: You're unsure of what is causing this issue, you have been previously fit and well. Your primary concern is the safety and care of your daughter, though feel you can't leave as an ambulance was sent for you and you would feel guilty. You expect that the hospital should take into account your daughters situation, which isn't really your fault, and be seen by someone who knows what to do as quickly as possible.

PMH: Asthma
DH: Prev IVDU + cannabis
SH: Ex-smoker, no OTC drugs, minimal alcohol intake

TOP TIPS

➕ Some scenarios will already have an established outcome and no matter how good your communication skills are you may not be able to alter this.

➕ Don't get frustrated, rather try to build rapport and see if you can gently come to a compromise.

COMMUNICATION

2.14 Refusal of Treatment

Scenario

You are the general surgery SHO on call at 7pm. You have been asked to speak to Miss Harris, a 28-year-old woman who was admitted earlier that day with suspected appendicitis. Her white cell count is raised, she has a temperature of 38.3°C and right iliac fossa tenderness with a positive Rovsing's sign; the surgical registrar has spoken to her already regarding having a laparoscopic appendicectomy that evening although she has not yet been consented. She has been commenced on IV co-amoxiclav. She has asked to speak to a doctor as apparently she does not want an operation.

How would you begin?

Introduce yourself and role, and establish what she knows so far.

You: "Hello Miss Harris my name is Dr. X I understand that you would like to speak to me. Could I begin by asking what has been explained to you so far?"

❝ **Patient:** "I've just been told that they think I have appendicitis and I need to have an operation to remove it tonight! Its all a bit much, can't I just see how I go with antibiotics?"

How will you respond?

Try to build rapport and show empathy while seeing if you can offer some further information.

You: "I understand its all a bit quick and confusing. Would you like me to explain to you what the operation involves?"

❝ **Patient:** "Well, I'm not sure I want one, I'll be in for days won't I? I need to be at home!"

You: "Usually most cases of appendicitis are treated and discharged within two days. It is a general anaesthetic, but it is a keyhole operation and usually only three small scars. Most people will go home the next day."

Try to explore the patient's ideas, concerns and expectations regarding treatment.

You: "Is there any particular reason why you are so anxious to get home?"

❝ **Patient:** "I only gave birth a week ago and my baby daughter is at home with my mum. This is the first time I've been away from her overnight, so I'd really rather not stay if I don't have to."

You: "Okay I understand that would be very worrying for me too. I would still recommend having the operation however as antibiotics may not sort this problem out and you may end up having a longer stay. What I can do is talk to the sister on the ward, and see if we can try to get you a side room so that you may be able to see your daughter more often."

COMMUNICATION

What would you do next?

Try to provide the patient with an explanation regarding the treatment to aid her understanding

You: "Would you like me to go through the procedure?"

66 **Patient:** "Yes please."

You: "After the anaesthetic doctor puts you to sleep, we will put three small cuts in your tummy to create ports. Using a camera, we have a look inside the abdomen, and then remove your appendix. The operation usually takes around one hour."

66 **Patient:** "OK, well that doesn't sound too bad."

How would you close the consultation?

You: "Do you have any questions?"

66 **Patient:** "Not at the moment thank you. I feel happier going ahead with the operation now it's been explained. I am just anxious to make sure my daughter is OK."

You: "Well I can give you some time to think things over and then I can come back and go through the consent form with you if that's okay?"

66 **Patient:** "Yes that's fine thank you."

SUMMARY

This again is a relatively straightforward scenario. The main issue here and that the patient is worried for her daughter and feels that the operation may delay her discharge. She is obviously not have the full procedure fully explain to her, and is also very anxious. The main points here are to give as much information as possible in the given time, explore her ideas, concerns and expectations so you can gain maximum points, and also come up with a possible compromise that may get the patient onside.

☺ Actor Brief

You are a 28-year-old woman who is feeling unwell and is very anxious. You have been told uou have appendicitis and need an operation tonight and then the doctor left. You have no idea what is going on!

Presenting Complaint: You are normally fit and well and are 8 weeks post partum. You had an uncomplicated pregnancy and normal vaginal delivery, with a healthy girl. You have been having some generalised abdominal pain for the last 3 days, a bit of diarrhoea yesterday and vomited once. You woke up this morning feeling sweaty, and were tossing and turning all night. You used your daughters' thermometer which showed a temp of 38°C. You saw your GP who sent you straight into hospital with no explanation why.

ICE: You have never been away from her before and are extremely anxious to be with her (she is currently with your mother)

PMH/DH/SH: Nil, uncomplicated delivery.

Special Instructions: You can be rather stubborn in your refusal until the procedure is explained.

TOP TIPS

➕ If the patient has capacity you must accept their decision even if you think it is unwise

➕ Offer your medical advice but do not be judgemental and show empathy and build rapport

➕ Don't worry if the patient still refuses treatment at the end of the scenario, this might be part of the actor's instructions

COMMUNICATION

2.15 | Post-Op Bile Leak

Scenario

You are the CT2 on the ward. Your patient is Mrs. Adams; a 34-year-old lady admitted for acute cholecystitis that has been treated with an emergency laparoscopic cholecystectomy. She has a BMI of 45 and the surgery was technically difficult. She is now five days post-op and has had a difficult recovery. She has had increasing pain in the right upper quadrant with general malaise and anorexia. A CT scan was performed and has shown suspicion of a bile leak and Mr. Stewart, your Consultant, has made the decision to return to theatre to explore the leak.

You have washed your hands and introduced yourself. Please explain the complication to the patient.

How would you begin the consultation?

Open the conversation by asking the patient what has happened to them so far and ascertain how much they know and understand.

You: "Hello Mrs. Adams, my name is Dr. X, I'm one of the doctors on the surgical team. I understand that you have recently had a scan and I am here to discuss the results with you. Before we go any further could I just ask you to tell me in your own words what has been happening over the past few days since the operation?"

66 **Patient:** *"Well, I was having all this trouble with my gallbladder so Mr. Stewart took it out last Monday. It was keyhole surgery and he said that I should be able to go home pretty quickly afterwards, but I've been on the ward feeling worse and worse for the past few days. I still have a lot of pain in the area and I just feel awful. I had the scan this morning to see what's wrong."*

What would you ask next?

Explain that you are here to discuss the scan results and the plan of action.

You: "I have looked at the scan results with Mr. Stewart and it appears that there has been a leak from the bile system. This is a complication that can sometimes happen with gallbladder surgery. I will explain to you what this means and what we are plan to do about it. Is that OK?"

66 **Patient:** *"Yes, I really want to get to the bottom of this pain. You say there is a complication from the surgery? That's very worrying. Mr. Stewart seemed like a competent surgeon, what's gone wrong?"*

How will you respond?

Explain that the frequency of complications is low. You can reassure the patient that this is not a case of surgical incompetence and that this is a recognised, although unfortunate, complication. You can say sorry to the patient; this is not an 'admission of guilt' but an important part of empathising with the patient.

You: "These complications are recognised but rare, happening in around 0.5% of patients who have this operation. When we need to do the operation as an emergency, as with your case, this can increase the risk. Mr. Stewart is a very experienced surgeon but sometimes we cannot predict these events. I'm sorry that this has happened in your case. I'd like to explain to you what we think has happened and what we plan to do about it."

66 **Patient:** *"Okay..."*

How would you explain the complication?

For this it is best to briefly review the patient's understanding of the operation. If you can draw a diagram that is clear this can be very helpful, but if your drawing skills are a bit rusty do some practice before the exam or don't take this approach as a bad diagram can confuse matters further!

You: "Did someone explain the operation to you beforehand?"

66 **Patient:** *"Yes, but that was last week and I can't remember all the details."*

You: "OK, I'll go over it for you and draw a diagram. The liver makes bile and this is stored in the gallbladder, which is fixed under the liver. There is a tube that drains from the liver into the bowel. A tube draining the gallbladder joins onto the one draining the liver. When we take out the gallbladder we need to cut the gallbladder tube and preserve the liver tube. Sometimes when we go in there is a lot of swelling and things are inflamed and stuck down, as in your case. We make every effort to see both tubes and only cut the gallbladder one. That being said, not everyone's anatomy is the same and the tube position can vary from person to person. What we think has happened is that the tube draining the liver has been damaged during the operation and has been leaking bile into your belly, making you feel unwell."

66 **Patient:** *"Oh, I see. So what does that mean?"*

Explain the plan to return to theatre

Explain that the management for the problem in this case is to return to theatre for another operation. This can also be done 'keyhole' and will likely require the insertion of a drain.

You: "In order to fix the leak we will need to do another surgery. This will be another keyhole procedure and we will likely put in a drain. This drain is a small plastic tube that goes from the bile duct to the outside world, through the skin here and drains the bile into a small bag. This diverts the bile and allows the damaged area to heal. I will speak to Mr. Stewart and come back later to explain the operation to you in more detail."

66 **Patient:** *"So this means I have to go and have another anaesthetic and another operation?"*

You: "Yes, I'm afraid so. We would aim to take you to theatre first thing tomorrow morning"

66 **Patient:** *"Alright, I understand what needs to happen."*

COMMUNICATION

How would you continue the consultation?

The patient could have various questions at this point in the consultation, the below would be some to anticipate. Remember, honesty is the best policy, if you do not know something do not lie. You can offer to go away and information-gather and come back to the patient with answers.

You: "Do you have any questions?"

" Patient: *"How much longer am I going to be in hospital? I wasn't expecting to be in so long."*

You: "You will need to be in hospital for at least a couple of days after the operation, but it is difficult to predict. The length of time that the drain needs to stay in is very variable, however some people go home with the drainage tube in place and come back for checks and to have it removed."

" Patient: *"Are there risks of more complications with further surgery?"*

You: "There are always risks associated with surgery and Mr. Stewart will be better placed to talk to you about the possible complications of this operation."

" Patient: *"What if I decide I don't want any more operations? Can we not just leave it alone to get better?"*

You: "Before you decide I'd like to make sure you have all the available information. At the moment there is bile leaking form where it should be into your belly. Bile is a digestive juice and will continue to make you feel very unwell and could result in you becoming even more unwell if we leave it. Unfortunately there are no medicines we can give that will fix it and it will not just heal if we leave it alone. You will always be able to make the final decision however surgery is the only way to fix this problem."

" Patient: *"You say that these complications can happen and that Mr. Stewart is very experienced, but what will your team be doing to make sure this doesn't happen to people in the future? I've had such a terrible time. I'd also like to know how to make a complaint. The ward staff have been very nice but I feel like this shouldn't have happened to me and I want to make a formal complaint to the hospital."*

You: "Whenever complications happen in surgery we discuss them at a large meeting every month, so that all the surgeons, from very experienced to new trainees, can learn from them. We go over the case and see if there was anything that could have been done differently.
I'm sorry things have not gone well for you. If you would like to put in a formal complaint this can be done though our Patient Liaison Service, and I can get their contact information for you."

How do you close the consultation?

You: "I'll come back later with Mr. Stewart. If you have any family you'd like to contact I'd be happy to explain what has happened if you'd like me to. If you have any other questions or need anything in the meantime the nursing staff can contact me on my bleep."

COMMUNICATION

Before leaving make plans for the next contact. This patient will need to consent to the operation after they have had it fully explained to them. Offer to do anything practical that you are able to before you leave, such as optimising analgesia or clarifying starving instructions for the morning.

SUMMARY

The focus of a station like this can vary; reassuring an anxious patient, dealing appropriately with an angry patient, facilitating a complaint, demonstrating effective explanation skills and demonstrating empathy. It could involve some or all of these aspects.
As with all communication stations always ensure that the environment is optimised, that you have quiet bleep-free space to see the patient, that a Nursing colleague can be present as well as anyone that the patient would like to be present e.g. spouse or family member.
You will come to the consultation with an agenda; to inform of the news, to explain what this means and to explain the next management steps. Beyond this the consultation will be led by the patient and you will need to answer their questions. Don't forget that communication is not just what you say but how you say it; you must convey the correct information in a professional but empathic way. Using drawing as part of your communication skills can be highly effective, so practice this before the exam.
In these scenarios the closure of the consultation will be determined by the patient. If they continue to ask questions then you have not yet answered everything in a satisfactory manner. If the mood escalates to anger you need to sensitively calm things.

COMMUNICATION

😐 Actor Brief

Mrs. Adams is a 34-year-old baker who was admitted several days earlier with right upper quadrant pain for 24 hours. This was treated with a cholecystectomy on the same admission. You were told you could go home soon after but have been getting further pain in the same area after the gall bladder was removed. You signed a consent form but didn't really pay attention to any risks.

Special Instructions: The actor should ask to make a complaint and once it is revealed that she will need to go back to surgery for a further operation.

TOP TIPS

➕ Make sure you address both your own agenda and the patient's in this scenario. You need to provide adequate explanation as well as answer their questions. Drawing diagrams can be useful and always check understanding.

➕ If the patient would like to complain you should be non-judgmental and assist them by signposting. It is best to be empathic but remain impartial.

2.16 Cancelled Operation

Scenario

You are an orthopaedic SHO assisting in an elective operating list. The list is over-running from multiple delays due to staff shortages and limited beds in recovery. The final patient on the list is Caroline Smith who is due to have a right knee ar-throscopy. It is 5:45pm and you have been asked to explain to her why her opera-tion has been cancelled. You have washed your hands and introduced yourself.

How would you begin?

You should start with general questions to establish what her understanding is and allow her to express her concerns

You: "Hello my name id Dr. X, I am from the surgical team. Can I confirm that you are Caroline Smith and that you have come today for keyhole surgery on your knee?"

> 66 **Patient:** *"Yes I have, my knee has been getting more painful over the year. I was cancelled a few months ago and haven't been able to work much since."*

What would you do next?

Continue to gather more information about the actor/patient as this will help address her concerns later in the consultation

You: "What work do you do? Why was the operation cancelled last time?"

> 66 **Patient:** *"I'm a postwoman and I've been off work since my knee has been playing up. I received a warning letter last week from my manager saying I had exceeded my maximum sick leave allowance. The operation was cancelled because the consultant had to be called away for an emergency. I didn't receive another date for 3 months."*

What would you ask next?

You can now break the bad news that the operation has been postponed. You need to clearly apologise and remember to offer to get them something to eat and drink

You: "I am very sorry to say that due to delays in theatre we will be unable to carry out your operation today. I understand that this is the second time you have been cancelled and that this is unacceptable. I will make sure that your operation is rescheduled for the earliest possible slot. Can I get you anything to eat and drink as I know you have been starved all day?"

> 66 *Patient [very angry]: "I feel dizzy because I haven't eaten all day I don't understand why my operation has been cancelled?"*

You have a duty of candour to explain that the operation was cancelled due to delays in theatre. You can say that you can avoid this happening next time by trying to get her operation scheduled earlier on the list. You can reassure her that the cancellations of operations are investigated by the hospital.

You: "Again I am very sorry that this has happened and I completely understand your frustration. We are also very frustrated. The booking office will rearrange your operation as a priority and they will also try to get you positioned earlier on the list to avoid this from happening again."

66 **Patient:** *"Why don't the staff just stay a bit later as this is only a short operation?!"*

Apologise that this is not possible and explain that it is not recommended that elective operations be performed outside working hours.

You: "Unfortunately that is not a possibility as the staff work set times beyond which we are not able to operate."

66 *Patient [demanding]: "When will my operation be rearranged?"*

Explain that the operation will be rescheduled to the next available slot but unfortunately you cannot give an exact date without liaising with the consultant and theatre co-ordinator.

You: "As I mentioned it will be re-arranged by the booking office as a priority."

66 **Patient:** *"I want to be given a date or at least a rough time period today and I will not leave until I have received this"*

Apologise and explain that it is unlikely that the theatre co-ordinator or booking office are available at this time. In urgent, non-emergent, trauma cases you might be able to bring the patient back the following day. Do not offer a time frame as you are not aware of the theatre slots available but reassure the patient they will be treated as a priority. You might also want to say that you will discuss the matter with the consultant and see if there are any other lists she can be put on.

You: "I do not have the precise information available at present but the booking office will inform you of the specific date and the operation will usually be within the next few weeks. The booking office will ring you within the next few days to confirm things. I will also discuss this with my consultant to see if there are any extra lists available so that we can get to you more quickly."

66 **Patient:** *"Can you guarantee that this will not happen again"*

You cannot guarantee that this will not happen again but you can reassure her that you will highlight that this is the second time she has been cancelled to reduce the chance of it happening again. You can try to put her early on the list to reduce the risk of cancellation from theatre delays.

You: "I can't offer any guarantees but we will try to prioritise your operation as much as we can as we really want to get things sorted for you."

66 **Patient:** *"I've had to spend a lot of money organising child care. Can I get this refunded? Who is going to pay for this next time?"*

Apologise for the additional cost but explain that unfortunately you cannot offer a refund or pay for childcare. You can offer that she discuss the situation with the Patient Advice and Liaison Service (PALS)

You: "Again, I am very sorry for the inconvenience caused. I can't advise you regarding child care but if you would like to take things further you can speak with the Patient Advice and Liaison Service (PALS)."

66 **Patient:** *"What about my work? Will my knee get worse if I walk on it?"*

Explain that significant weight bearing activity (such as delivering mail) may increase the wear on the knee. However, she should continue to be active and continue non-weight-bearing excise, such as swimming, to keep her knee muscles strong. You can offer to refer her to physiotherapy and optimise her analgesia.

You: "You should continue as before the operation. As mentioned we will try and get you back in as soon as possible so this should minimise any further disruptions. Weight-bearing shouldn't cause significant damage but your knee will continue to be sore."

66 **Patient:** *"My work are saying that I will lose my job unless I go back!"*

You can offer to write a sick note explaining that the operation has been cancelled and that she is unable to carry out an active job. You can suggest that she contacts her union for support and to get advice on the terms and conditions for sick leave.

You: "I am sorry to hear this. I can provide you with a medical sick note to say you cannot perform your current duties if you feel unable to because of your knee. You might want to see if you can come to a compromise in work so that you can perform light duties or other roles while your knee is hurting."

66 **Patient:** *"Well I just want to go now. I hope you can get me back in as quickly as possible."*

You: "I am sorry again for the cancellation and we will endeavour to get you back in as soon as possible."

SUMMARY

Cancellation of an elective operation on the day is reported as occurring in 1% of cases in 2014/15. This can occur due to clinical and non-clinical reasons. Common non-clinical reasons for cancellations include; theatre lists over-running; staff unavailable; emergency case needing theatre; admin error; critical care bed unavailable. The cancellation of elective operations 'on the day' for non-clinical reasons is addressed in the Handbook to the NHS Constitution which states that

"All patients who have operations cancelled, on or after the day of admission (including the day of surgery), for non-clinical reasons should be offered another binding date within 28 days, or the patient's treatment be funded at the time and hospital of the patient's choice"

If a patient is offered a reasonable date within 28 days but prefers to be treated later then this does not apply. Patients may also be suspended from the waiting list for clinical reasons if they are unfit for the procedure.

🙂 Actor Brief

You are Caroline Smith, a 27 year old who presented with a 3 month history of knee pain and locking. You work as a postwoman and the knee pain is so bad you have had to have time off work. It is now getting toward the time when your employer will no longer pay you for time off. You were expecting to have your operation today and have been fasting since midnight. It is now 5:45pm and so you are very keen to get it over with. You previously had an operation cancelled as the consultant was called away on the day and there was a clerical error meaning that it took 3 further months before this operation date.

PMH: Nil

DH: NKDA, Nil regualr

SH: Lives with boyfriend, smokes socially

Special Instructions: You should act understandably frustrated when the candidate explains the operation has been cancelled. If they deliver the news particularly badly, give them a bit of a hard time.

TOP TIPS

➕ This station puts you in a challenging situation and the actor will only respond positively if you are able to listen to her concerns and show empathy towards her situation

➕ The questions become progressively more difficult and bring up problems, such as child care issues, where you may be unable to offer definitive solutions.

➕ The actor will likely respond positively if you are pro-active in offering suggestions such as writing a sick note, getting her early on the list, referring to physiotherapy and offering her something to eat and drink.

COMMUNICATION

2.17 Angry Relative: Dislocated THR

Scenario

You are the covering on call Orthopaedic registrar. The nursing staff inform you that Mr. Smith's daughter is adamant she would like to speak to a doctor regarding the surgical care of her father who has dislocated his hip two weeks post op. The patient has just been transferred to theatre for a manipulation under anaesthetic of his right hip.

You have entered the patient's room to discuss the treatment and management plan with the patient's daughter.

How would you begin?

Introduce yourself, and begin with an open question to allow the relative to explain as much as she feels able to. Try not to interrupt and actively listen to the history.

You: "Hello, my name is Mr. X, I am part of the surgical team. Can I confirm your name and relationship to Mr. Smith? I understand you had some questions regarding your father's surgical treatment?"

❝ **Daughter:** *"I have been quite worried following this admission as I was told that my father's new hip should resolve all his symptoms. Was there a problem with the surgery itself and will this same problem manifest in the future?"*

What would you ask next?

You should continue to gather information. It is too soon to use close questions as you may miss something important. Use a further open question to give the actor/relative another opportunity to disclose information.

You: "Do you have any other concerns regarding the current management plan?"

❝ **Daughter:** *"Well I am concerned that the initial surgery had not gone exactly to plan. I was also told he may need a new hip in 10 or 15 years, is this true given the current situation?"*

What would you ask next?

As the relative seems to have offered all that she is going to now would be a good time to explore her ideas, concerns and expectations (ICE). These should again be open questions to give the actor/relative the opportunity to divulge more information.

You: "What do you think is going on? What is your main concern? What were you expecting when you came here today?"

❝ **Daughter:** *"I have been quite worried that my father's hip has either broken or dislocated. He is very frail and suffers from several medical conditions and I fear he may not tolerate repeated surgeries like this in the future. I am also concerned there is no one at home to look after him when he is discharged. I was hoping for* *ideas to help prevent this situation happening in the future and also perhaps some help with my father's care at home."*

Now that you know the actor/relative's main ideas, concerns and expectations regarding the consultation you can proceed onto focused, closed statements to help you explain to the relative what was happened. Ideally this should be done in a structured format referring to a timeline of events.

You: "Your father had an unwitnessed fall at home which most likely resulted in a twisting injury of the right hip. This has caused a hip dislocation as excessive strains of movement had been placed on the prosthetic hip. The dislocation had been confirmed by imaging and there was no associated fracture. "

Daughter: *"Well what happens now?"*

You: "The most important plan of action at this point is to transfer your father to theatre and relocate the hip. This can be easier to perform in theatre as general anaesthetic is often needed to relax the muscles around the hip to help with the relocation and provide sufficient pain relief. After this we will mobilise him with the physios and he will be able to go home when safe."

Daughter: *"Is this because the operation was not performed correctly then?"*

You: "Unfortunately one risk of performing a hip replacement is a dislocation. This often happens when the movement in the hip is stretched beyond its normal plane. The relative risks of this happening are quite rare however in certain circumstances such as an awkward fall such symptoms can present. This does not necessarily mean that the surgery itself was performed incorrectly and on the table, after the new hip is put in the prosthetic joint is tested in all planes of movement to assess stability. Hips are more prone to dislocating in the first 6-8 weeks following surgery as the muscles and tissues around the hip joint heal and that is why certain movements are restricted by the physios. As this was a fall I suspect your father has just been unlicky.""

Daughter: *"What are the chances it will dislocate again?"*

You: "The risks of having another dislocation in the future are raised slightly following this first dislocation. However as we are still within the first 6-8 weeks and the muscles are healing and your father has fallen there is nothing to say that the hip itself is unstable. We would only be concerned if it dislocated after this period and then it might require a revision procedure to replace the hip."

What else would you like to explore?

Once you are happy that you have fully explained the potential reasoning behind the dislocation and the subsequent management plan, you can briefly discuss social options available to the patient following discharge. Of course you can redirect the patient and her relative to the relevant health care professional to discuss these issues in greater depth.

You: "Is there anything else you concerning you?"

Daughter: *"I still don't feel like Dad is coping well at home. Is there anyone who can give him some more help?"*

You: "The occupational therapists are key members of the health care team. They can carry out home assessment including re-enablement packages to help identify any care issues when the patient has returned to their home environment and can suggest various modifications including stair lifts etc. They can also suggest a social package of care which includes carers coming to the home to help with general activities of daily living e.g. administering medication. Prior to your father's discharge he will be introduced to an occupational therapist."

How would you close the scenario?

You: "To summarise we will take your father to theatre and relocate the hip as soon as we have some theatre space. We will then mobilise him with our physios and have the occupational therapists assess him before we let him go home. We will then see him back in our clinic at the routine 6-8 week mark to see how he his doing. Is there anything else you think I have not covered?"

66 **Daughter:** *"No that all sounds fine, thank you again."*

SUMMARY

Your consultation should focus on exploring the concerns the patient's relative has and exploring them in a structured format through a timeline of events.

Prosthetic hip dislocation is a rare risk that may occur following surgery. This is minimised by assessing degree of stability of the hip intraoperatively as well as stringent physiotherapy regimen to attempt to strengthen the muscles around the hip joint.
One of the common surgical emergencies following hip dislocation includes nerve impingement and vessel laceration. Hence a full neurovasculature assessment needs to be conducted and the patient transferred to theatre in a timely fashion.

It is important to quantify the risk of a repeat dislocation occurring in the future however explain that at risk patients will have more stringent surveillance and follow up to prevent this from happening.

😐 Actor Brief

You are Alice Roberts, daughter of Mr.. Roberts – a 65-year-old gentleman who has been admitted following a fall at home. He now complains of painful hip and is unable to weight bear. There are suspicions he may have dislocated his hip. You are concerned given it is only two weeks since his operation for a total hip replacement that this has happened.

Presenting Complaint: You are concerned about the nature of the initial operation, whether something had gone wrong to result in your father's hip dislocating. There is concern that this might happen again and you are unsure what can be done to prevent this.

ICE: You are concerned about your father's health and his ability to tolerate repeated anaesthetic procedures. You also feel some extra help at home is warranted given your father's deteriorating health and reduced mobility.

TOP TIPS

➕ After using open questions your information gathering closed questions should focus on the future management plan and social care

➕ Remember to show empathy. The actor/relative is clearly a concerned daughter who is worried about her father

➕ Involving other members of the healthcare team can be a useful tool to explore some of her social concerns regarding discharge

COMMUNICATION

2.18 Smoking Cessation

Scenario

Mr. Goyal has been referred to your Vascular outpatients clinic on a 'as soon as' basis by a conscientious GP who feels he has significant peripheral arterial disease in his right leg.

You have washed your hands and introduced yourself. Please take a history for 5 minutes and then counsel the patient on the effects of smoking and smoking cessation.

How would you begin?

You: "Hello Mr. Goyal. I'm Dr. X. Your GP has asked me to see you about your legs. Can you tell me what's been going on?"

Patient: *"Well doctor, I've got to be honest, I almost didn't come today – I'm supposed to be doing a run up to Scarborough and the boss isn't taking it well but my GP was pretty insistent I show up and get checked out. My legs have been giving me a bit of gyp recently."*

What will you ask next?

Continue to gather information using another open question but with a little more focus on the key symptoms.

You: "I see, and how have your legs been bothering you exactly?"

Patient: *"Well they hurt a fair bit of the time and this has been going on for a good few years, especially when I walk a lot, or go uphill. I've been managing OK, I just stop and wait for it to settle then carry on but over the past few months it's been getting worse. Now I even notice it at night and end up getting up to shake it off although having my feet over the edge of the bed helps a bit. It's mostly my right leg to be honest. It's making me tired and I can't risk being tired on the job."*

What will you ask next?

Now is a good time to assess the patient's ideas, concerns and expectations and also to use closed questions to identify any modifiable vascular risk factors.

You: "You mentioned your job, it sounds like that's important to you - what is it you do?"

Patient: *"I'm a lorry driver but my boss doesn't take to kindly to people having sick days often, I can't afford to take too much time off".*

You: "I can understand that's obviously a big worry for you then" (Empathy!) "I'd like to ask a few more questions about your legs/health. Do you ever get pain in your legs/feet when you're sitting for example watching TV?"

Patient: *"No, it's only when I walk and then like I said, at night in bed."*

You: "And how far can you walk before they start hurting?"

66 **Patient:** *"Oh about 100 yards, but less uphill."*

You: "Do you have any other medical problems?"

66 **Patient:** *"Just a bit of high blood pressure, surgery for a hernia and asthma."*

You: "Do you smoke?"

66 **Patient:** *"I smoke around 30 cigarettes a day and have done so for the last 30 yrs."*

You: "Do you drink alcohol?"

66 **Patient:** *"Not heavily, maybe around 1 or 2 pints of beer a few times a week when I'm not working the next day."*

What would you do now?

Having identified the risk factors and key components of the vascular history together with the patient's concerns you may now deliver information in the form of smoking cessation advice.

You: "Mr. Goyal, I'd like to talk to you about smoking and trying to quit. Is that something you've ever tried to do or considered doing?"

66 **Patient:** *"Yeah yeah, I know it's bad for me, but so are lots of things. I tried to quit a few times but only managed a day here and there. I know someone who's gran lived to 98 and smoked like a chimney so it can't do that much harm."* (Patient has unrealistic ideas based on an outlier – every smoker knows someone who was a smoker who lived to be very old). Yeah I have a bad chest but no offence that's not what I'm here for."

You: "Actually Mr. Goyal, unfortunately smoking affects more than just your lungs and breathing. Smoking is one of the biggest risks for developing blocked blood vessels. The symptoms you've told me about suggest you have blocked or partially blocked blood vessels in your legs, especially your right side. I'll take time to explain what needs to happen next but first can we discuss you quitting smoking again?"

66 **Patient:** *"Really?! Blocked vessels? I mean I know it's bad for me to smoke but I had no idea it affected my legs. Will I be able to continue working?"*

You: "The work issue depends on different factors which we can come on to in a moment. How do you feel about quitting?"

66 **Patient:** *"I guess I could give it another shot. Will it make my feet better?"*

COMMUNICATION

You: "It is unlikely to but it will slow down or halt the vessel disease getting any worse for the time being. Ultimately with this kind of vessel disease there is a very real risk you could lose your foot. Quitting smoking will greatly improve your chances that this doesn't happen."

66 **Patient:** *"Lose my foot!! Really? I don't even know where to begin quitting. Last time I tried it didn't work, but I didn't even have patches or anything."*

You: "Well I'd like to write to your GP and get them on board with supporting you quitting and prescribing patches, would that be OK?"

66 **Patient:** *"Yes, thank you, I can book in with my GP this week, my boss won't like it but I'm gonna need help if I'm going to quit. I can't lose my foot!"*

(Unfortunately most consultations about smoking cessation in reality are not this easy or successful, nor is there sufficient GP infrastructure to holistically support would-be quitters but perseverance and educating the patient are key).

How would you close the consultation?

You: "Mr. Goyal, as I understand it you've been suffering with this leg pain, especially your right foot, for the past few years but it has worsened recently to the point where it is interfering with your sleep. Walking, especially uphill aggravates the pain while rest helps. Having your feet hanging down is also useful. You're worried about holding onto your job and as we've discussed your smoking habit is a big part of what's going on with your feet and their blood supply. We will need to arrange further imaging to see if there are any blockages of the blood vessels running to your feet."

SUMMARY

This history should convince you that Mr. Goyal has impending critical limb ischaemia and requires further investigation. He will ultimately likely need a bypass procedure (or angioplasty).
Peripheral vascular disease is very common, especially among smokers. There are many lifestyle factors that increase the risk of disease. Between 55-70 around 1 in 20 to 1 in 10 people have a degree of peripheral arterial disease. Over 70, 1 in 5 will have peripheral arterial disease. Of all patients, 1 in 5 will go on to develop critical limb ischaemia. Of these, 1 in 4 will go on to have an amputation.
This patient is a typical vascular patient with many risk factors and will likely head on to have an amputation of his foot if he does not implement lifestyle changes, appropriate antiplatelet therapy (aspirin and/or clopidogrel) and ultimately will need further imaging CT or MRI angiography to quantify his vessel disease. Duplex scanning can be also used but in this patient's case MRA would be more appropriate-as a guideline CT is useful for iliac disease while MRI is useful for SFA/distal blockages as it is better at visualising small vessel disease.

Smoking cessation is an important aspect of a clinical encounter. It is easy as a clinician to become 'jaded' with smokers and cease advising them to stop smoking however if even one quits as a result of your advice, their health and the burden on the NHS will be better for it. Identifying at what stage they are at in their decision making is key: Pre-contemplation, Contemplation, Planning, Action, Reinforcement. Once you know where they are mentally with respect to their habit your aim is to move them to the next stage.

COMMUNICATION

😐 Actor Brief

You (Mr. Goyal) are a 47-year-old lorry driver who smokes 30 cigarettes a day since 14 years old. You are an overweight single man who spends most of your time on the road. Your GP has referred you to Vascular Outpatients on a 'urgent' basis as a new referral because of right foot pain.

Presenting Complaint: You have started to get increasing calf pain when you walk any distance, especially uphill. This first started about 3-4 years ago but recently over the past 2-3 months you have found that increasingly at night you get pain in your legs, especially your right foot/calf, and end up hanging your feet out the end of the bed or getting up and walking about in order to help the pain settle. Painkillers don't really work. There is no ulceration of your legs but they do stay quite cool most of the time. You notice your feet turn red when they hang over the edge of the bed. You finally went to your GP a couple days ago and they arranged an urgent appointment for today.

ICE: You're worried about being able to continue working. In fact you're already worried about missing work to come to this appointment and have only come because the pain has gotten so bad that it's interfering with work.
You think their will be some new medication that will 'sort out' the foot pain.

PMH/DH/SH: Hypertension, high cholesterol, 'asthma' (actually COPD), your GP has been recently checking your blood sugars and they are a bit high – the GP has told you it could be diabetes starting, previous appendicectomy, inguinal hernia repair. Allergic to penicillin. Not very compliant with medications for hypertension, not on any antiplatelet therapy. You smoke 30/day for the past 33 years. 1-2 pints of beer a few times/week. You live alone in a bedsit on the third floor. FHx Father had 'bad legs' and died of a heart attack.

Special Instructions: You generally are dismissive of your health and do not link smoking (which in your mind affects the lungs) with vascular disease without sufficient explanation from the doctor.

COMMUNICATION

TOP TIPS

➕ Establish the patient's attitude to smoking. Have they thought about quitting? Tried before? If they haven't you need to adjust your advice accordingly.

➕ Make sure you understand the physiology of atherosclerotic disease. If you do not, trying to explain this in lay terms to someone else will sound vague and unconvincing.

➕ Limb loss should not just be used as a shock tactic for smoking cessation. It is a genuine possibility in a critically ischaemic limb and needs to be appropriately raised and discussed.

2.19 Jehovah's Witness

Scenario

You are the general surgical SHO on call. You have been asked to see Mrs. Jones on the surgical admissions unit who had been admitted earlier that day following a large PR bleed. The haematology lab has called the ward with the results of her most recent blood tests, which show her current haemoglobin is 66. She is not actively bleeding and is haemodynamically stable. She is a known Jehovah's Witness and has already mentioned to the FY1 who clerked her that she does not want a blood transfusion.

Her admission clerking and most recent blood tests observations and are available for you to review in this station. You may make notes on the paper provided to take with you to the next station. In the next station you will be asked to speak with Mrs. Jones. Please do not take the patient notes with you.

You have 1 minute reading time then a 9 minute prep station then a 10 minute communication station with an actor.

🖉 Documents

Admission clerking – FY1

78 year old lady
- Fresh PR bleed earlier today with abdon pain
- no recent change in bowel habit, no weight loss.
- no previous history of PR bleed
Pt is Jehovah's Witness
PMHx: Hypertension
DHx: NKDA, Bisoprolol
O/E: Apyrexial, non-tender abdomen, PR: fresh blood on glove
Imp: ? Haemorrhoids ?ischaemic colitis ?diverticular disease
Plan: IVI, Fluid balance, NBM, Snr R/V on WR.

Blood Results: Hb 66, all otherwise normal
Drug Chart: Simple analgesia written up. 1 bag of Hartmann's stat given in A&E.
Obs Chart: BP138/62 HR88 RR18 Sats 96%

How would you begin?

Begin with an open question.

You: "Hello my name is Dr. X and I am one of the surgical team. Is it Mrs. Jones? What have you been told so far?"

> 66 **Patient:** *"Nothing really, doctor. I came in with this bleeding from my back passage. Everyone's been very nice but all they've done is take some blood tests, I just don't know what to think."*

What will you do next?

From this you know that the patient is aware that blood tests have been taken. She appears slightly distressed despite reassurance and so it is important to explore her ideas, concerns and expectations.

You: 'What is concerning you most at the minute?'

❝ **Patient:** *"Just all this bleeding. It was terrifying! All over the toilet!"*

You: "Is there anything else that is worrying you?"

❝ **Patient:** *"Actually, yes. When I asked the doctor what bloods she was taking she said there was one for transfusion. I am a Jehovah's Witness and this is not acceptable. I know I have lost a lot of blood but will not have a transfusion under any circumstances."*

What will be your next steps?

The patient has directly expressed a wish not to have a blood transfusion.

You: "I apologise that she took a sample for blood transfusion without your consent, we will take your wishes into account. We have now got back the results of your recent blood tests, and it does show that your haemoglobin level is very low."

❝ **Patient:** *"I don't care, under no circumstances will I have a transfusion."*

At this point, it is important to make sure that the patient is fully aware of the choice she is making and possible adverse outcome.

You: "I understand however I just need to make sure that you understand that having a low blood count can be a very serious problem, and there is a risk that you could die from this."

❝ **Patient:** *"Yes I do understand that."*

What will you ask next?

Although Mrs. Jones has declined a blood transfusion, many Jehovah's Witnesses will accept derivatives of blood components. Her opinion on this must be explored.

You: "You have told me you would not have a blood transfusion. There are other products available that we can give. Do you know anything about these? If so what are your thoughts?"

Jehovah's Witnesses are often very well educated on the options available to them. If this is the case, she may well know what she is happy to consent to. If not, you must provide her with the relevant information. You could also offer to contact the local Hospital Liaison Committee for Jehovah's Witnesses representative to discuss her options.

❝ **Patient:** *"Yes I had to do some research on this when my husband was in hospital a few years ago. I do not what blood products in any form and am well aware of the consequences of my decision."*

COMMUNICATION

What would you do next?

This is not a decision that you should be taking on your own. It is important that you inform the Consultant whose care she is under, and following this, it would be advisable to discuss with the haematologist. You should let the patient know you will do this.

You: "I respect your wishes surrounding a blood transfusion. Just to let you know I will need to inform the consultant who is looking after your care about your decision and he may also wish to come and talk to you himself. I can also get you some more information on the alternative options available to you if you wish?"

66 **Patient:** *"Yes please, I would appreciate that."*

What options could be available to a patient?

• Iron and other vitamins
• Albumin
• Recombinant clotting factors
• Prothrombin complex concentrate
• Firbrinogen concentrate
• Acute normovolaemic haemodilution
• Fibrin glues and sealants

SUMMARY

This can be a very sensitive issue and needs to be approached with caution, remaining respectful of the patient's decision and non-judgemental throughout. Patients' capacity and full understanding of the risks of declining the transfusion need to be explored, as well as the extent of their knowledge of the options available to them.
Jehovah's Witnesses refuse blood transfusions, including autologous transfusions in which a person has their own blood stored to be used later in a medical procedure, (though some Witnesses will accept autologous procedures such as dialysis or cell salvage in which their blood is not stored) and the use of packed RBCs (red blood cells), WBCs (white blood cells), plasma or platelets.

Cell-free blood products, containing haemoglobin but not red blood cells have recently become available and may be acceptable for some Jehovah's Witnesses.

Although Jehovah's Witnesses cannot accept blood, they are open to other medical procedures. Jehovah's Witness Hospital Liaison Committees maintain lists of doctors who are prepared to be consulted with a view to treatment without the use of blood transfusion. This has eased many of the tensions related to the issue.

In 2000 the Witnesses changed the rules on blood transfusions so that the Church would no longer take action against a Witness who willingly and without regret underwent a blood transfusion. Some people wrongly interpreted the change as meaning that Witnesses could now accept blood. But the actual change was just that the Church would not take disciplinary action against that Witness.

😐 Actor Brief

You are Mrs. Jones, a 78-year-old lady who has presented with a large volume PR bleed. You are very anxious about being in hospital.

Presenting Complaint: You woke up this morning with a generalised stomach ache. You went to the toilet and found that, mixed with your stool was a large quantity of bright red blood. You have never noticed anything like this before.

Significant PMH/DH/SH: You take a tablet for your blood pressure but otherwise fit and well. You are a Jehovah's Witness and do not wish to have a blood transfusion, even in life threatening circumstances.

TOP TIPS

➕ It is important to explore fully Mrs. Jones' wishes and not just presume that she does not want any treatment for her low haemoglobin levels.

➕ Don't be judgmental or feel you need to persuade her to do well at the scenario. Rather offer her the available options and encourage her to discuss things with her relatives and local Witness committee.

COMMUNICATION

2.20 Transfer of a Patient

Scenario

In this station you will have a set of patient notes to read. You will then move to the next station where you will be asked to phone a colleague and discuss the patient with them.

You are the general surgical CT2 on call in a DGH. You have just taken handover from the out-going SHO who did not have time to refer Mrs. Green to the local vascular centre. You have not seen the patient but you have her notes and recent results available to review. You may make your own notes on the paper provided. In the next station, you will phone the on-call vascular consultant at the local centre.

Documents

Admission clerking – Surgical FY2
Admitted 1 day ago
72 year old lady
- 4 day history of left lower abdominal pain and diarrhoea.
- no change in bowel habit, no blood, no mucus, no weight loss.
- felt feverish during the last 24 hours
PMHx: Hypertension, previous appendicectomy (years ago), occasional angina (on walking quickly),
DHx: Amlodipine, Aspirin, GTN spray PRN, Lactulose. NDKA
O/E: Pyrexial 38.1, tender but no guarding LIF
Imp: Diverticulitis
Plan: Abx, IVI, Fluid balance, NBM, Snr R/V on WR.

Today 08:45: WR Mr. Zed, consultant general surgeon
Hx ncted.
Imp: Likely diverticulitis
Plan: Continue current management
             CT abdo/pelvis
             Colonoscopy when well.

Today 18:45: Surgical FY1
ATSP Re: pain left arm
Sudden on-set pain in left arm. Cool, some tingling. Painful arm.
Feels heavy. First noticed discomfort at 1600.
O/E: Cool left forearm compared to right.
Patient able to move fingers.
Decreased sensation.
Radial and ulnar pulses not felt.
Capillary refill 4s.
Plan: Analgesia
             Senior review.

COMMUNICATION

Obs charts: Pyrexia on admission which has now settled. Tachycardia 130bpm on admission, now 100 bpm. Other obs unremarkable. Last observations charted at 1600.

Admission ECG: Atrial fibrillation

Bloods: Raised inflammatory markers (WCC and CRP), mild improvement on repeat bloods.

How would you begin?

It is important to try and maintain a structure in order to transfer the appropriate information efficiently. A useful framework to start with is SBAR (situation, background, assessment, recommendation):

Situation
You: "Mr. Ray, my name is Dr. X., I am the CT2 on call at DGH. I am calling you regarding a 72 year old lady with an ischaemic arm."

66 **Vascular Consultant:** *"OK, what's happened?"*

Background
You: "She has a background of AF and originally presented septic, with abdominal pain and diarrhoea. She is currently in under the care of Mr. Zed with suspected diverticulitis."

66 **Vascular Consultant:** *"So what do you think is going on?"*

Assessment:
You: "She complained of a painful left arm at 4pm and on examination has a cool left arm with reduced sensation and no palpable pulses, We feel she has an ischaemic limb secondary to an acute embolic event."

66 **Vascular Consultant:** *"And you want to transfer her over here?"*

Recommendations:
You: "I feel this lady needs an urgent vascular review and a possible embolectomy to restore blood flow to her left arm."

What will you ask next?

66 **Vascular Consultant:** *"I agree. Sounds like we've got to see her. Get her blue-lighted across and we will expect her."*

You: "Is there anything else you'd like us to do prior to transfer?'

66 **Vascular Consultant:** *"Whatever you feel is sensible but don't delay getting her over to us."*

You: "OK, I will inform the bed managers. In the meantime I will arrange a repeat ECG and observations and initiate treatment for AF as appropriate."

Vascular Consultant: "Great. I'll pass you to my reg who will take the details."

SUMMARY

SBAR is used in this situation to deliver the relevant information to the consultant in a structured fashion. There is quite a bit of information but you should stick to the most important facts. Clearly this lady has had an acute vascular event and it is important you confidently give the consultant a summary of the clinical details. It is also important that you clearly state the reason for calling. In this instance you feel the patient needs to be transferred.

😐 Actor Brief

You are Mr. Langford, the on-call consultant vascular surgeon at Doctorsville General Hospital.

You receive a phone call from an SHO a CT2 at the local DGH. They are calling you regarding a patient with an ischaemic limb. This patient is at risk of losing a limb therefore you advise that she gets blue-lighted to your A&E where you will see the patient as soon as possible.

Special Instructions: You are tired and stressed. It is 9pm on Sunday. You have had a particular busy weekend on-call and have been operating all day. Your wife has just rung to say your daughter is unwell and she is taking her to A&E.

TOP TIPS

➕ Read the information given to you carefully. Even though you have not personally seen the patient you will still be expected to have thorough knowledge of the case.

➕ DO NOT LIE about having seen the patient. The examiner knows the brief, and knows you have not seen them yet *(however improbable this may seem in reality!)*. You will lose significant points for making up information.

➕ The aim of this scenario is to ensure you can deliver information effectively in order to ensure patient safety. Only provide relevant information, and deliver it in a clear and concise manner. Answer questions honestly.

COMMUNICATION

3 HISTORIES

3.1 | Change In Bowel Habit

Scenario

Your next clinic patient is Fiona Harrison. She is a 34-year-old lady who has been referred to your lower GI clinic with a change in bowel habit over the last six weeks.

You have washed your hands and introduced yourself. Please take a history and suggest a management plan.

How would you begin?

Begin with an open question and allow the patient to explain as much as she feels able to. Try not to interrupt and actively listen to the history.

You: "Can you tell me what has been going on?"

66 **Patient:** *"I have been quite worried as over the last few months I have been having trouble with my bowels. I am usually very regular but last month I was quite constipated and now I have had a few episodes of diarrhoea."*

What would you ask next?

You should continue to gather information. It is too soon to use close questions as you may miss something important. Use a further open question to give the actor/patient another opportunity to disclose information.

You: "Have you had any other symptoms?"

66 **Patient:** *"Well I think I might have passed some blood as there was blood on the toilet paper but I thought this was because I was straining. Other than that I can't think of anything really."*

What would you ask next?

As the patient seems to have offered all that she is going to now would be a good time to explore her ideas, concerns and expectations (ICE). These should again be open questions to give the actor/patient the opportunity to divulge more information.

You: "What do you think is going on? What is your main concern? What were you expecting when you came here today?"

66 **Patient:** *"I have been quite worried as my father died from bowel cancer in his early 40s and I remember he had lost weight. I'm a single parent, my daughter is only four and I'm worried how I will manage if there is something seriously wrong. My GP told me you would want to do some tests"*

HISTORIES

What questions would you ask that might lead you to a diagnosis?

Now that you know the actor/patient's main ideas, concerns and expectations regarding the consultation and have given her ample opportunity to tell you about the history of her condition you can proceed onto focused, closed questions to help you make a diagnosis.

✎ Focussed Bowel Habit Questions

You will want to know the exact onset of symptoms and what the symptoms actually are. In particular you want to know:
• Has she noticed any weight loss/does she think her clothes are looser than normal?
• How often/many times a day is she opening her bowels?
• Is she getting abdominal pain?
• Is the pain intermittent/colicky/constant or relieved by defecation?
• Has she had any mucus or blood PR?
• Have her symptoms progressed?
• Has she felt tired or had any non-specific symptoms suggestive of anaemia?
• Has her appetite changed?
• Has she noticed any extra-intestinal symptoms such as swollen lymph nodes, eye problems, ulcers or anything associated with inflammatory bowel syndrome?

"" Patient: *"Now that you mention it I have lost around 2 stone in weight over the last 2 months but I have been dieting and exercising. I have always had occasional abdominal pains as my GP told me I have IBS. The pain at the moment is usually in the left side. At the moment I am opening my bowels around 5 times a day and it is watery. I think it's probably got worse over the last few months. I feel otherwise well, I have a good appetite."*

What else would you like to ask?

Once you are happy that you fully understand the presenting complaint and the patient's concerns you should quickly run through the rest of the history to double check that you have not missed anything that could be relevant. You should cover PMH, DH, SH and a quick systems review.

You: "Do you have any other medical conditions?"

"" Patient: *"I have IBS."*

You:
"Do you have any allergies?"

"" Patient: *"No, just cats."*

You: "Do you take any medications?"

"" Patient: *"I used to take mebeverine for my IBS but I don't take it anymore."*

You: "Do you smoke or drink?"

Patient: *"I know I shouldn't but I smoke around 20 cigarettes a day, only Marlboro lights though!"*

You: "What do you do for work? Who is there at home with you?"

Patient: *"I'm a solicitor and it's just me and my four year old at home."*

You: "Is there anything else that you have noticed that we haven't mentioned yet?"

Patient: *"No everything else is fin, my eyes hurt occasionally but I'm waiting to get my glasses changed."*

How would you close the scenario?

Now that you have come to the end of your history it is good practise to summarise back to the patient to ensure you have all the facts. This also allows her the opportunity to add/ correct anything. After summarising you can check there is nothing else she wishes to add before thanking her and explaining what your management plan is.

You: "You have been opening your bowels 5-times per day over the last 2-months which was preceded by episodes of constipation. You have lost around 2 stone in weight over this time and have noticed blood in the stool with intermittent left-sided abdominal pain. Is this correct or is there anything else you think I have missed?"

Patient: *"No that is everything."*

You: "From what you have told me there could be a number of things causing your symptoms. Given your family history we want to exclude the most serious conditions such as colon cancer. Before we definitely know what is causing your symptoms we need to request some tests. I would like to get some blood tests and an X-Ray in the first instance. The gold standard test for establishing what is going on in your bowel involves passing a tube with a camera into your bowel through the back passage in our endoscopy suite. This allows the endoscopist to look at the bowel wall and to take pictures and biopsy any areas of concern. I would then like to see you back in clinic and we can discuss where we go from there. Do you have any questions?"

Patient: *"No, that all makes sense. How soon will the tests be?"*

You: "Given that we want to exclude possibility of a cancer the scope will be listed as urgent, this will prioritise the procedure and it should happen within two weeks. You will get a letter in the post or a phone call explaining where and when you need to attend."

Patient: *"OK, that makes sense. I don't think I have any further questions at the moment. Thank you."*

HISTORIES

SUMMARY

Your history should focus on the onset of symptoms, progression of symptoms and highlight red flag symptoms such as weight loss, PR bleeding, symptoms of anaemia or positive family history.

Inflammatory bowel disease (IBD) is a group of inflammatory conditions of the colon and small intestine. Crohn's disease and ulcerative colitis are the principal types of inflammatory bowel disease.

Irritable Bowel Syndrome (IBS) is a functional bowel disorder characterized by more than 6 months of recurrent abdominal pain/discomfort, which may be relieved by defecation and associated with an alteration in stool form or frequency. Consider in those with abdominal pain, bloating and change in bowel habit.

In the United Kingdom '2-week' and 'urgent' referrals are defined by the following criteria:

2 week wait referral criteria:
• Definite palpable right-sided abdominal mass (to exclude caecal tumour)
• Definite rectal mass of PR exam
• Unexplained iron deficiency anaemia with:
- Hb<11g/dl in men
- Hb<10g/dl in non-menstruating women
• 40-60 yrs old with persistent (> 6 weeks) rectal bleeding and a change to looser/more frequent stools
• 60 yrs or over with persistent (>6 weeks) rectal bleeding (in the absence of anal symptoms) and/or change to looser/more frequent stools

Urgent referral:
• Rectal bleeding in the absence of anal symptoms/haemorrhoids
• Blood mixed with stool and or clots
• Rectal bleeding and associated change to looser stool (any age)
• Unexplained weight loss
• Strong family history of colorectal cancer. (1st degree relative with colorectal cancer <50 yrs old or 2 1st degree relatives with colorectal cancer at any age)
• Iron deficiency anemia

😐 Actor Brief

You are Fiona Harrison a 34-year-old lawyer; you are a single-parent with a four-year-old daughter. You are very nervous about attending the clinic as your father died of bowel cancer.

Presenting Complaint: You have had around 2 stone in weight loss over the last 2-months. You had been dieting but you can't seem to keep any weight on. You have noticed that you are opening your bowels 4-5 times per day and you have noticed blood in the stool. Prior to this you had some episodes of constipation but these have now resolved.

ICE: You are not sure what is going on but you are worried that it might be bowel cancer as your father died of this aged 44. You want to be sent for an urgent scan.

PMH/DH/SH: You smoke 20 cigarettes per day are recently divorced and have no other health problems.

TOP TIPS

➕ After using open questions your information gathering closed questions should focus on red flags for change in bowel habit

➕ Remember to show empathy. The actor/patient has a young child and is a single parent

➕ Did you spot that she mentioned eye pain? Anterior uveitis is associated with HLA-B27 conditions such as Crohn's disease and her smoking makes her more at risk of Crohn's than ulcerative colitis.

HISTORIES

3.2 | Back Pain

Scenario

You are the night on call SHO for Trauma and Orthopaedics and are asked by ED to assess Miss Tiffany Brocklehurst, a 24-year-old female who is morbidly obese with severe back pain. Please take a history and suggest a management plan.

How would you begin?

You: "Hello Miss Brocklehurst, I'm Dr. X, can you tell me what's troubling you?"

66 **Patient:** *"Oh doctor, I'm in agony, my back, it's so sore! And my leg! It's terrible. I normally have a very high pain threshold but this is so bad."*

What would you ask next?

You: "I'm sorry to hear you're in so much pain. Really sounds like you're struggling. Can you tell me more about how this all started?"

66 **Patient:** *"Well I went to pick up my son off the floor earlier this evening to stop him crying and I got this sudden pain in my lower back. It shot down my right leg. I couldn't move and my Mother had to call the ambulance. It took the two ambulance men and my Dad to get me off the floor onto the stretcher. It was agony! I told the nurse earlier, the pain is 11/10!"*

What would you ask next?

Now is a good time to identify the patient's idea, concerns, and expectations.

You: "I can obviously see you're in pain. Is there anything else about this that is worrying you?"

66 **Patient:** *"Oh doctor, I have had back pain before, but never this bad. I know when I saw the back doctor a few years ago he said that there was no surgery options but surely I need an operation to fix this?!"*

You: "Miss Brocklehurst this is clearly very upsetting for you. I'd like to ask some more questions before we discuss what options are available if that's all right?"

66 **Patient:** *"OK doctor."*

What questions would you ask that might lead you to a diagnosis?

Now that you know the actor/patient's main ideas, concerns and expectations regarding the consultation and have given her ample opportunity to tell you about the history of her condition you can proceed onto focused, closed questions to help you make a diagnosis.

You: "You said the pain was 11/10 and shooting down your right leg, did the pain move anywhere else?"

66 **Patient:** *"No, just the middle and sides of my lower back and down my right leg."*

You: "What kind of pain was it?"

66 **Patient:** *"Shooting stabbing pain."*

You: "Does anything make the pain worse?"

66 **Patient:** *"Any movement doctor, walking is almost impossible."*

You: "Have you tried any painkillers"

66 **Patient:** *"Well the nurse gave me something here and that's helped, but barely. I didn't take anything at home because I didn't want it to mask my problem so you could assess me properly."*

You: " I'm sorry you're in pain. I'll arrange for the nurse to give you some more pain killers in a moment. May I just ask some specific questions to assess if your spinal cord is affected."

✏️ Focussed Back Pain Questions

You will want to know the exact onset of symptoms and what the symptoms actually are. In particular you want to know:
• Any leg or foot weakness? No
• Any change in the sensation of your back/legs? Yes my Right leg is tingling, like pins and needles and my foot feels a bit numb.
• Any saddle anaesthesia? (Do not ask in this manner. Ask something like have you noticed any numbness when you are wiping yourself after going to the toilet?) No
• Any incontinence? (Again, ask if they have soiled or wet themselves if they don't know what you mean.) No
• Any painless urinary retention? (Ask if they can feel when their bladder is full/can they tell that they need to pass urine?) Yes I can feel my bladder is full and I know when I need to use the toilet.
• Any night pain? No worse than the day pain.
• Any recent infections like a chest infection, water work infection? No. (Can seed infection into disc but not a likely differential in this case).

What else would you like to ask?

You: "Do you have any other medical conditions?"

66 **Patient:** *"I have IBS and asthma."*

You: "Have you had any operations in the past?"

66 **Patient:** *"Yes I had my gallbladder out 2 years ago."*

You: "Do you have any allergies?"

66 **Patient:** *"No I don't doctor."*

You: "Do you take any medications?

66 **Patient:** *"I use my inhalers daily and take co-codamol most days as it helps with my back pain normally."*

You: "Do you smoke/drink?"

66 **Patient:** *"I smoke 20-30 a day. But some days I only smoke about 15. I'm trying to cut down. I don't often drink any alcohol – I'm too busy looking after my kids."*

You: "Who's at home with you?"

66 **Patient:** *"I live with my Mum and Dad and my two little ones, Chaz and Toby."*

You: "And lastly are you currently in work or a full-time mum?"

66 **Patient:** *"I work part-time in a nearby care home as a carer."*

How would you close the scenario?

Now is a good time to summarise back to the patient and to clarify what has been said before suggesting a management plan.

You: "Miss Brocklehurst, thank you for answering my questions. Just so I make sure I've got everything may I go over everything? As I understand it you have struggled with back pain for the past 6 years but tonight you had much more severe pain when bending down to pick up your son. You do not have any weakness in your legs and have not noticed any numbness around your genitals. You have control of your bladder and bowels and have not had any accidents – you can feel when your bladder is full. You have however experienced severe pain across your back and down your right leg and have also experienced pins and needles/numbness in your right leg. Is there anything else you would like to add?"

66 **Patient:** *"No, that's exactly it doctor."*

You: "My main differential would be disc prolapse with muscle spasm and sciatic symptoms on the right side however I would like to fully examine the patient including a spine exam, neurological exam and DRE to assess anal tone/sensation. Important differentials to exclude would be cauda equina syndrome, possible infection of the disc and malignancy."

Following clinical examination what investigations or tests would you order to aid your diagnosis?

You: "Following examination I would want to know the patients vital observations including temperature, take blood tests to check for infection/inflammation, a urine dip to check for a UTI, a pre and post void bladder scan to check for painless retention and if there were any worrying features or uncertainty of diagnosis I would want to order an MRI of the patient's lumbosacral spine on an urgent basis to assess any compromise to the cauda equina."

SUMMARY

Your history should focus on the onset of symptoms, progression of symptoms and high-light red flag symptoms such as painless urinary retention, urinary/faecal incontinence, saddle anaesthesia, leg weakness/paraesthesia.

Most acute back pain patients are not cauda equina but to miss such a diagnosis is unacceptable. It causes permanent disability/impaired quality of life for the patient and on a Trust level it is indefensible in court – resulting in the trust being sued and large sums being paid to the patient affected. Cauda Equina Syndrome is reasonably rare – incidence roughly 1 in 33,000 to 1 in 100,000. Ideally patients with CES should be undergoing surgical decompression within 24 hours of onset of symptoms. (Cauda equina syndrome: a review of the current clinical and medico-legal position. Gardner et al. Eur Spine J. 2011 May; 20(5): 690-697)

Lower back pain in general is a huge socioeconomic burden. In 2014/15 employees took 2, 957, 000 days of sick leave in the UK and there were 223,000 new cases in 2014/15. Certain occupations have a higher incidence of lower back pain, especially construction and caring personal services.

🙂 Actor Brief

You are Tiffany Brocklehurst, you are 24 years old, morbidly obese and come from a British travelling family. You live in a caravan park outside of town.

Presenting Complaint: You were bending down to pick up your 3 year old son earlier this evening when you felt severe back pain that radiated down your right leg. You were then unable to move and your ma called the ambulance. It has not abated despite the ED nurse giving you painkillers and the pain shoots down your right leg. You also feel like the top of your foot is a bit numb.

ICE: You want the pain to go away. You think that surgery will fix your back for good despite previous consultations where you were told that surgery is not the answer.

PMH/DH/SH: You've had chronic back pain for 6 years ever since you had your first child but never as severe as this episode. You also have asthma, IBS and underwent a cholecystectomy 2 years ago. You are morbidly obese, NKDA. You use regular inhalers and co-codamol for your back pain. You smoke 20 cigarettes per day, rarely drink alcohol. You live with your parents and your two children aged 6 and 3 in a caravan park. You work as a part-time care assistant at a local care home.

Special Instructions: You are melodramatic, your pain is "11 out of 10", you are not good with pain (despite you thinking you are) and you are keen to remain in hospital for the night. You also want surgery as you think this will make everything go away.

The doctor needs to mention weight loss as part of their management plan, this is acceptable. If they are rude or dismissive in broaching this sensitive topic become hysterical and accuse the doctor of calling you fat.

TOP TIPS

➕ Acute on chronic back pain, especially in melodramatic patients is often tedious and time-consuming. The mainstay of treatment is reassurance, analgesia, lifestyle advice and patient education, none of which are the quick fixes the patient wants/expects but do not be tempted to cut corners – always screen thoroughly for cauda equina and spinal abscesses *(if they're known to pain clinic they may well have had a spinal injection)* or malignancy.

3.3   Anxiety and Palpitations Pre-Op

Scenario

You are a general surgical registrar preparing for an elective theatre list. You are asked by a nurse to review a 30-year-old lady who has attended for an elective laparoscopic cholecystectomy but has been having palpitations. You have washed your hands and introduced yourself. Please take a history and suggest a management plan.

How would you begin?

Although palpitations are usually benign, they may be associated with a potentially life-threatening cardiac disorder. Therefore it is important to start by saying that you would assess the patient and ensure she was stable following an ABC approach as per ALS guidelines. You should stress the importance of getting an immediate 12 lead ECG. Once you have established that she is stable you can start a history using open questions

You: "Can you tell me what has been going on?"

Patient: *"I've been getting palpitations on and off for the past 4 months, they only last a few minutes and then settle down. I think it is probably caused by stress as I'm a bit worried about the operation today."*

What would you do you next?

You should continue to gather information. 'Palpitations' can mean a number of different things in colloquial speech and you should clarify exactly what the patient means. Use a further open question to give the actor/patient another opportunity to disclose information.

You: "Please tell me more about your palpitations?"

Patient: *"It feels like my heart is leaping out of my chest and I feel a bit light headed. They come on particularly when I'm tired or at night when I'm going to sleep and worrying about work."*

You: "Can you tell me about any other symptoms you've had?"

Patient: *"I have been a bit more tired than usual and I'm working long hours. My job is very stressful at the moment and I have to drink a lot of coffee to keep me awake at work. My bowels have also been a bit more loose and I get tummy cramps probably because of the coffee!"*

What questions would you ask that might lead you to a diagnosis?

Now that you given her ample opportunity to tell you about the history of her condition you can proceed onto focused, closed questions to help you make a diagnosis.

HISTORIES

> ### ✎ Focussed Anxiety and Palpitation Questions
>
> You want to know:
> • Nature of the palpitations: Are her palpitations fast or slow? Do the palpitations come on gradually or suddenly? How long do they last? Is there anything that triggers the episodes (e.g. exercise, stress or coffee)? Has she ever tried stopping the palpitations by holding her breath?
> • Does she get any shortness of breath, chest pain or light headedness
> • Has she noticed feeling hot or cold?
> • Has she had any changes in and/or appetite
> • Has she noticed any change in bowel habit
> • Has she had any changes in her menstrual cycle?

Patient: *"The palpitations are fast, come on suddenly and last about 15 minutes. I've lost about 1 stone in the last two months but haven't been trying to diet. I've also been feeling quite hot and have to sleep on top of the bed covers at night. My periods have been a bit irregular for the last couple of months and I've been meaning to see my GP but didn't have the time due to work."*

What else would you like to ask?

Once you are happy that you fully understand the presenting complaint and the patient's concerns you should quickly run through the rest of the history to double check that you have not missed anything that could be relevant.
• Past medical history including history of asthma as β agonists can cause sinus tachycardia. In addition ask about previous cardiac/cerebrovascular disease and psychiatric illness such as anxiety disorders
• Drug history: There are a number of drugs which can cause palpitations including β agonists, theophylline, macrolide antibiotics, domperidone and recreational drugs (cocaine and amphetamines).
• Family history: Any family history of sudden cardiac death or hypertrophic cardiomyopathy which can present with palpitations and sudden death due to VT
• Social history: Ask more about alcohol and caffeine intake and smoking

You: "Do you have any other medical conditions? Do you have asthma or any previous problems with the heart?"

Tip - these questions have been listed here, but in reality you would ask them individually and wait for an answer before asking the next.

❝ **Patient:** *"I have gallstones and I used to have IBS. The tummy cramps I've been getting remind me of my IBS symptoms. I don't have asthma or heart problems."*

You: "Do you take any medications?"

❝ **Patient:** *"I'm taking microgynon."*

You: "Do you have any family history of heart problems?"

❝ **Patient:** *"No."*

You: "How much coffee do you drink? Do you smoke/drink?"

❝ **Patient:** *"I have to drink about 8-10 cups a day. I have never smoked and I drink a couple of glasses of wine a week."*

You: "Is there anything else that we haven't mentioned that you feel is important?"

❝ **Patient:** *"No everything else is fine, I have a dull pain at the back of my eyes and I'm going to see an optician."*

How would you close the scenario?

Now that you have come to the end of your history it is good practise to summarise back to the patient to ensure you have all the facts. This also allows her the opportunity to add/correct anything. After summarising you can check there is nothing else she wishes to add before thanking her and explaining what your management plan is.

You: "Just so I know I've understood anything let me summarise, and if there's anything I've missed please let me know. You have been having sudden onset rapid palpitation for the last 4 months. This has been associated with fatigue, weight loss, heat intolerance, loose stools, stomach cramps and irregular periods. Is this correct? Is there anything else you think I have missed?"

❝ **Patient:** *"No that all sounds right."*

Explain your management plan to the patient

It is important that you clearly explain your plan and the reasons why her laparoscopic cholecystecomy should be rescheduled

You: "From what you have told me there could be a number of things causing your symptoms but the most likely is an overactive thyroid gland. There are other potential causes and we need to investigate these also, before we proceed. Without knowing what the cause is it is not safe to proceed with the operation today, so unfortunately we need to postpone the operation. We will do some blood tests today to check your thyroid and we also need an ECG to monitor your heart rate. Based on the results of these tests, I will ask either a thyroid specialist or heart doctor to see you to start treating these causes."

The patient does not want her operation cancelled and asks for the blood tests to be performed immediately and if normal proceed with the operation. What do you say next?

Tip - You should show empathy but also be assertive. When patients become upset or angry in a situation such as this, you must remember that you are acting in the patient's best interests. It is not safe to proceed with an elective operation under any circumstances and you should not allow yourself to do so. You must however, avoid an argument and destroying doctor-patient relationship.

You: "Clearly you've been waiting some time to get this done and it can be hugely frustrating and upsetting when something like this halts progress. I'm sorry but it's just not safe to proceed without knowing what's going on and for that we need to do a number of tests and wait for the results. One investigation you'll need is heart monitoring for at least 24 hours. Without these tests it is dangerous for you have general anaesthetic."

What is your differential diagnosis?

- Hyperthyroidism with signs of thyrotoxicosis
- Tachyarrhythmias such as SVT, atrial fibrillation or atrial flutter
- Drugs: Palpitations secondary to caffeine intake, beta agonists
- Psychiatric: Anxiety disorder
- Physiological: Pregnancy
- Rare: Phaeochromocytoma

Following clinical examination what investigations would you order to aid your diagnosis?

- Thyroid function tests, FBC, U&Es, Calcium
- Thyroid auto-antibodies: Anti-TSH receptor antibodies and Anti-thyroid peroxidase antibodies
- Resting 12-lead ECG and ambulatory ECG: A 24-hour ECG may needed
- Echocardiography to exclude structural heart disease
- US neck if any features of goitre
- Chest x-ray

SUMMARY

Graves disease is the most common cause of hyperthyroidism in the UK. It is an immunological disorder caused by thyroid-receptor antibodies or immunoglobulins stimulating TSH receptors to secrete T3 and T4. Patients often present with a variety of symptoms including palpitations, weight loss, heat intolerance, bowel frequency and Oligomenorrhea. The diagnosis is confirmed by the presence of ophthamomopathy which is characteristic of Graves' disease. It is caused by autoantibody damage resulting in orbital fat swelling. Initial treatment would include carbimazole or propylthiouracil to inhibit thyroid hormone production and return the patient to a euthyroid state. She must be warned of the risk of carbimazole induced neutropenia and to stop the drug immediately if she develops any symptoms. Beta-blockers can also be used to control symptoms. Many patients are now treated with radioiodine as a single oral dose. Surgical treatment is reserved for patients with large goitres or if there are contraindications to radioiodine. Contraindications to radioiodine include pregnancy, breast-feeding or contact with young children.

😐 Actor Brief

You are Ami Smith, a 30 year old, financial analyst in the city. You have just started a new job and are working very long hours. You believe the palpitations are down to anxiety and do not want your lap chole to be cancelled as you've been on a long waiting list and don't want to take more time off work.

Presenting Complaint: You have had palpitations for about 4 months. These are sudden onset and last about 15 minutes. They occur particularly when you go to bed. You have lost 1 stone in weight over the 2 months without any dieting and you are quite pleased about this. You have noticed that you have been feeling very tired at work and quite hot at night. Your bowels have been loose and you have been getting stomach cramps. You have noticed a dull pain in the back of your eyes and your periods have also been irregular.

PMH/DH/SH: You drink 8-10 cups of strong coffee a day at work

Special Instructions: If the candidate says that operation should be cancelled try to persuade them to change their mind. Request that the tests are done immediately and then the operation could be done later in the day.

TOP TIPS

➕ The history should cover not only the nature of palpitation but also the other systemic features associated with hyperthyroidism.

➕ Try to be empathic but assertive as the patient will try and persuade you that this is simply anxiety and her operation should not be cancelled.

3.4 Progressive Dysphagia

Scenario

Your next clinic patient is Louise Hyde. She is a 74-year-old lady who has been referred to your upper GI clinic with a change in bowel habit over the last six weeks.
You have washed your hands and introduced yourself. Please take a history and
suggest a management plan.

How would you begin?

Begin with an open question and allow the patient to explain as much as she feels able to.
Try not to interrupt and actively listen to the history.

You: "What's brought you in today?'"

66 **Patient:** *"My GP sent me in. I saw him last week because I can't keep anything
down. I've been struggling to eat and drink for the last month or so and my daughter was worried because I'd lost so much weight."*

What would you ask next?

You should continue to gather information. It is too soon to use close questions as you
may miss something important. Use a further open question to give the actor/patient
another opportunity to disclose information.

You: "Can you tell me a bit more about the swallowing problem?"

66 **Patient:** *"It started a few months ago, I found it harder to eat things like chicken
and boiled potatoes. It seemed to stick in my throat and take a long time to go
down. I switched to soups and mashed potato but that became difficult too. Drinking was okay to start with but now I can only manage small sips and sometimes
even that makes me vomit. My husband thinks I've lost more than a stone."*

What would you ask next?

As the patient seems to have offered all that she is going to now would be a good time to
explore her ideas, concerns and expectations (ICE). These should again be open questions to give the actor/patient the opportunity to divulge more information.

You: "What do you think is going on? What is your main concern? What were you expecting when you came here today?"

66 **Patient:** *"I don't want to come into hospital. My GP told me you would want to do
some tests. But my husband has got dementia and I don't want to leave him at
home on his own."*

What questions would you ask that might lead you to a diagnosis?

Now that you know the actor/patient's main ideas, concerns and expectations regarding the consultation and have given her ample opportunity to tell you about the history of her condition you can proceed onto focused, closed questions to help you make a diagnosis.

🖉 **Focussed Progressive Dysphagis Questions**

You will want to know the exact onset of symptoms and what the symptoms actually are. In particular you want to know:
- Do you get any pain on swallowing?
- Does this happen every time you eat and drink or is it intermittent?
- Have you lost any weight?
- Do you have problems with heartburn or acid reflux?
- Do you ever cough after eating or drinking? Have you been treated for any chest infections recently?
- Have you noticed any voice hoarseness?
- Any blood in your vomit or stool?
- Are you still passing urine? What colour is it?
- Have you ever had this before?
- Have you had an OGD in the past?

❝ **Patient:** *"It's not pain as such, it just feels like an uncomfortable sticking sensation. Then I am sick, there is no blood in it. Now it happens every time I eat or drink anything. I've lost quite a lot of weight, I think about a stone over the last month or so. I used to get heartburn until my doctor started a tablet a few years ago. I've never had this before. I had a camera down into my stomach around 10 years ago but none since. My voice hasn't changed. Eating and drinking doesn't make me cough, it just all comes straight back up. I'm still passing small amounts of urine but it's quite dark. I haven't had any weakness in my limbs."*

What else would you like to ask?

Once you are happy that you fully understand the presenting complaint and the patient's concerns you should quickly run through the rest of the history to double check that you have not missed anything that could be relevant. You should cover PMH, DH, SH and a quick systems review.

You: "Do you have any other medical conditions?"

❝ **Patient:** *"No."*

You: "Do you have any allergies?"

❝ **Patient:** *"No."*

You: "Do you take any medications?"

❝ **Patient:** *"Aspirin and lansoprazole."*

You: "Do you smoke/drink?"

> 66   **Patient:** *"I've never smoked. I have a drink on special occasions."*

You: "What do you do for work? Who is there at home with you?"

> 66   **Patient:** *"I'm retired, I used to be a librarian. I live my husband, Bob, he's got early stage dementia, so I am his main carer. I've got one grown up daughter who lives 50 miles away."*

How would you close the scenario?

Now that you have come to the end of your history it is good practise to summarise back to the patient to ensure you have all the facts. This also allows her the opportunity to add/ correct anything. After summarising you can check there is nothing else she wishes to add before thanking her and explaining what your management plan is.

You: "Just to check I've not missed anything I will summarise what you've told me. Over the last month you have experienced difficulty swallowing first solids then liquids. You have lost around 1 stone in weight over this time and feel lethargic. You don't have any other associated features. You are otherwise fit and well and are the main carer for your husband. Is there anything else you think I have missed?"

> 66   **Patient:** *"No that all sounds right."*

What is your differential diagnosis?

In a 74-year-old female my differential diagnosis includes:
- Oesophageal carcinoma
- Oesophageal stricture
- Achalasia
- Extrinsic compression- lung cancer, retrosternal goitre
- Neuromuscular disorders- CVA, myasthenia gravis

Following clinical examination what investigations would you order to aid your diagnosis?

- Bloods- iron deficiency anaemia
- OGD + brushings/ biopsy
- Endoscopic ultrasound to assess wall invasion
- CT chest-abdo-pelvis- for staging

Please explain your management plan to the patient

It is important that you clearly explain your plan and while trying not to worry the patient unnecessarily. Given however, that you are suspecting that this may be cancer, you should be honest with the patient about this.

You: "From what you have told me there could be a number of things causing your symptoms. At this point I do not know what the cause is, but because your symptoms have progressed quickly, I have to consider some more sinister causes. Do you know what I mean when I say 'sinister causes'?"

> 66   **Patient:** *"No."*

You: "Like I said, we have to consider all the causes. For any symptoms we must consider the "common" causes, but we must also the consider the rarer causes that we should never miss. In this case our "never miss" cause is cancer."

66 **Patient:** *"Oh no! You think I've got cancer?"*

You: "At this point I don't know and that why I'd like to arrange some urgent tests to find out. Because you are unable to keep anything down I would like to do some blood tests, particularly to make sure you haven't become dehydrated and require admission to hospital. The gold standard test for establishing what is going on in involves passing a tube with a camera into your stomach through your mouth, it is the same test you had 10 years ago. This allows the endoscopist to look at the bowel wall and to take pictures and biopsy any areas of concern. I would then like to see you back in clinic and we can discuss where we go from there. Do you have any questions?"

66 **Patient:** *"Yes, that all makes sense. Thank you."*

SUMMARY

Oesophageal cancer most commonly affects male patients over the age 60. Adenocarcinoma followed by squamous cell carcinoma are the most common types. Adenocarcinoma tends to affect the lower oesophagus while SCCs affect the upper and middle thirds. Risk factors include smoking, alcohol excess, Barrett's oesophagus and achalasia.

Oesophageal cancer tends to present late and as such prognosis is generally poor, with a 12% ten year survival rate. It is staged using the TMN system. Treatment for stage 1 cancer is oesophagectomy or occasionally endoscopic mucosal resection. Stage 2-3 cancers can be down-staged with neoadjuvant chemotherapy followed by surgical resection. However, this depends on the fitness of the patient for extensive surgery. Stage 4 cancers are treated with chemo/radiotherapy and symptomatic control.

☺ **Actor Brief**

You are Louise Hyde a 74-year-old retired librarian. You have been sent in by your GP with difficulty swallowing solids and now liquids. You are worried about leaving your husband, Bob, at home alone as he has dementia.

Presenting Complaint: One month ago you began to find it difficult to swallow solid food, you noticed an unpleasant sticking sensation in your throat. You changed your diet to softer foods but now even liquids are coming back up. You have lost over one stone in weight and feel weak and tired. You are passing urine less often and in smaller volumes, and it is concentrated in colour. There have been no other associated symptoms.

HISTORIES

ICE: Your main concern is leaving your husband alone. You are worried that this could be something serious and are concerned about having lots of investigations and a prolonged hospital stay as you are his main carer.

Significant PMH/DH/SH: You have never smoked. You drink only at special occasions. You take aspirin but don't know why and your GP started lansoprazole around 5 years ago for heartburn. You had an endoscopy 10 years ago because of anaemia but were told it was normal. You live with your husband, Bob, who has early stage dementia who needs support with dressing and eating.

TOP TIPS

➕ Elderly patients with dysphagia and recurrent vomiting are at high risk of dehydration and AKI, some of these patients may need to be admitted for inpatient investigation and concurrent fluid therapy.

➕ It is useful to know the key 2 week wait criteria for common surgical malignancies.

HISTORIES

3.5 Neck Lump

> ## Scenario
> Your next patient is Claire Turner, a 34-year old lady. She has been referred to the head and neck clinic by her GP with an enlarging neck lump. You have washed your hands and introduced yourself. Please take a history and suggest a management plan.

How would you begin?

Begin with an open question and allow the patient to explain as much as he feels able to. Try not to interrupt and actively listen to the history.

You: "What has brought you here today?"

66 **Patient:** *"I've got this lump in the middle of my neck. I noticed it a few weeks ago, but recently I think I can feel another one in my neck too."*

What would you ask next?

You should continue to gather information. It is too soon to use close questions as you may miss something important. Use a further open question to give the actor/patient another opportunity to disclose information.

You: "Have you had any other symptoms?"

66 **Patient:** *"I've not felt well for the last two weeks, I've been very lethargic. I think it's because I've been waking up in the night sweating profusely. I have to have a cold shower to cool down."*

What would you ask next?

As the patient is in discomfort and therefore a concise historian, explore his thoughts briefly before focusing your questions.

You: "What do you think is going on? What is your main concern? What were you expecting when you came here today?"

66 **Patient:** *"I'm worried that it could be a cancer. Do you think it's cancer?"*

What questions would you ask that might lead you to a diagnosis?

Now that you his presenting complaint you can proceed onto focused, closed questions to help you make a diagnosis.

HISTORIES

✏️ Focussed Neck Lump Questions

- Do the lumps come and go or are they progressively getting bigger?
- Have you noticed any lump anywhere else?
- Any pain in your neck?
- Have you lost any weight?
- Have you noticed any change in your voice?
- Any swelling in your arms or legs?
- Have you had cough or cold recently?
- Have you been abroad recently?

❝❝ Patient: *"The lumps are getting bigger, they don't really hurt but sometimes ache. I haven't felt any other lumps. I've dropped a dress size, it must be because I'm constantly sweating at night. I haven't noticed a change in voice or any swelling in my arms or legs. I've had a runny nose but so has my daughter and it's settling now. I went to Tenerife 3 weeks ago."*

What else would you like to ask?

Once you are happy that you fully understand the presenting complaint and the patient's concerns you should quickly run through the rest of the history to double check that you have not missed anything that could be relevant. You should cover PMH, DH, SH and a quick systems review.

You: "Do you have any other medical conditions? Have you had any operations?"

❝❝ Patient: *"No, I'm normally well."*

You: "Do you have any allergies?"

❝❝ Patient: *"No."*

You: "Do you take any medications?"

❝❝ Patient: *"I don't take any medication."*

You: "Do you smoke/drink?"

❝❝ Patient: *"I've never smoked. I only drink at weekends, a bottle of wine or so with my friends."*

You: "What do you do for work? Who is there at home with you?"

❝❝ Patient: *"I work part time in a supermarket. I live with my husband and my 3 year old daughter."*

How would you close the scenario?

Now that you have come to the end of your history it is good practise to summarise back to the patient to ensure you have all the facts. This also allows him the opportunity to add/correct anything. After summarising you can check there is nothing else she wishes to add before thanking her and explaining what your management plan is.

66 **You:** *"You noticed a painless, progressively enlarging lump in your neck a few weeks ago, another neck lump has since developed. It is associated with night sweats and weight loss. You have no past medical history and don't take any medications. Is there anything else you think I have missed?"*

Patient: "No."

What is your differential diagnosis?

In a 34-year-old lady my differential diagnosis includes:
• Lymphoma
• TB
• Viral lymphadenopathy
• Metastatic disease

Following clinical examination what investigations would you order to aid your diagnosis?

• Bloods
• Lymph node biopsy: either ultrasound guided or excisional biopsy
• CT scan for staging

Please explain your management plan to the patient

You: "There are lots of causes for a lump in the neck and therefore we need to start with some simple investigations. I would like to examine your neck and lymph nodes first of all, then take some blood tests. In order to find out the nature of the lump, we need to take a small sample of tissue via a biopsy. This will involve injecting some local anaesthetic around the area to numb it before taking the sample. The tissue will then be looked at under the microscope, these results take around 2 weeks to come back. After the results are available, I will arrange to see you in clinic and we will take it from there. Do you have any questions?"

66 **Patient:** *"Could it be cancer?"*

You: "Some cancers such as lymphoma can present with a neck lump and night sweats. But there are also other common things that can cause a similar picture. The point of the biopsy is to identify the cell types in the lump and this will give us a better idea as to the cause, until then try not to worry and as soon as the results are available I will discuss them with you."

SUMMARY

In a young patient with a new neck lump, night sweats and weight loss, lymphoma is the most likely diagnosis.

HISTORIES

Lymphoma is broadly divided into two categories: Hodgkin's and non-Hodgkin's. Hodgkin's lymphoma tends to affect patients in their 20-30s while non-Hodgkin's is more common in those over 60 years.

Treatment largely consists of chemotherapy and radiotherapy. Hodgkin's lymphoma, despite being a relatively aggressive disease, has a good prognosis with a high cure rate. Non-Hodgkin's lymphoma is much more variable in treatment response due to the many different subtypes. It can be divided into low and high grade which determines prognosis.

😐 Actor Brief

You are Claire Turner, a 34 year old part time shop assistant. You developed a lump in your neck 3 weeks ago and saw your GP. You live with your husband and 3 year old daughter. You are worried that you might have cancer and have read about your symptoms on the internet.

Presenting Complaint: You noticed a small lump in the middle of your neck 3 weeks ago, since then it has increased in size. Last week you also noticed another lump to the left of your neck just above your collarbone. They are not painful but occasionally ache. This has been associated with night sweats drenching the sheets and you have to frequently get up during the night to have a cold shower. You have been very tired recently and are struggling to spend as much time as you sued to with your daughter. You have also gone from a size 14 to a size 12 in the last month without dieting.

ICE: You are frightened that you have cancer, you Googled your symptoms and lymphoma was the most frequent result.

Significant PMH/DH/SH: You work part time in a supermarket and live with your husband and 3 year old daughter. You have no allergies. You have no medical problems and take no medication. You have never smoked and drink a bottle of wine over the weekend but nothing during the week.

TOP TIPS

➕ An isolated neck lump has many differentials, it is often the lack or presence of associated symptoms that make the diagnosis clear. Therefore, a thorough but focused history is important.

➕ When asked 'could it be cancer?' It is important not to falsely reassure patients when the history is highly suggestive. Often outlining a management plan with clear follow up can help put them at ease whilst awaiting results.

➕ Explain your management plan as you would in clinic, outlining the steps clearly and when they can expect to see you again.

3.6 | Carpal Tunnel

Scenario

Your next clinic patient is Mr. Brian Wolfson, a 66 year old gentleman who presents with a tingling sensation in his right hand.
You have washed your hands and introduced yourself to the patient. Please take a history and suggest a management plan.

How would you begin?

Begin with an open question to establish the exact nature of the presenting complaint.
Tip: 'Tingling' can mean different things to different people and it is therefore important to elicit Mr. Wolfson's original testimony. Allow the patient to continue uninterrupted and show signs of active listening throughout.

You: "How can I help you today, Mr. Wolfson?"

> **Patient:** *"Well, doctor, I've come to see you because of this problem with my right hand. I get this weird sort of tingling that keeps waking me up in the middle of the night. I'm getting more and more tired and frustrated and just want to get to the bottom of what's going on and sort it out."*

What would you ask next?

Mr. Wolfson has given some helpful information regarding his expectations which you should remember for later, and thus demonstrate you were listening. At this point however, you need to elicit more information about the nature, duration and functional consequences of the presenting complaint. Ask another open question at this early point in the consultation.

You: "Well we will certainly do all we can to get to the bottom of this. For now could you please tell me a bit more about this problem?"

> **Patient:** *"Yes, of course. I suppose I first noticed the tingling about three months ago and it's got worse since then. It feels a bit like pins and needles – like when you bang your funny bone – and only affects my right hand. It comes and goes during the day but only becomes a big problem at night when it wakes me up."*

What else would you like to ask?

Mr. Wolfson has clarified what he means by tingling, describing a parasthesia rather than numbness or pain. He has also outlined the duration of this chronic and apparently progressive problem. You have not however, determined the exact site of the problem or identified any other troublesome symptoms, therefore it is now appropriate to ask more focused questions.
You: "Is the tingling across the whole hand or limited to specific fingers or your palm? Have you had any other problems with your right hand? Have you had any other symptoms?"

HISTORIES

Patient: *"Well, yes, the tingling is actually limited to my thumb, index finger and sometimes my middle finger. I've not felt it in my ring finger or pinky. I'd not really considered that before. My wife has also noticed I've been a bit more clumsy recently – knocking things over with my right hand, dropping cups of tea and the like. Other than that, I'm very well in myself."*

What else would you like to ask?

The patient has described a distribution of 'tingling' suggestive of a peripheral mononeuropathy. His associated clumsiness adds further evidence to support a specific pathology. You can now ask more focused questions about other associated symptoms to further refine your differential diagnosis, elicit Mr. Wolfson's ideas about the cause of his symptoms, and any associated concerns.

You: "Have you noticed any weakness in your thumb movements? For example, when you're holding a pen or gripping a steering wheel?"

Patient: *"No, I haven't had any problems with weakness; my writing has been unaffected, and the same with driving."*

You: "Have you had any ideas about what might be causing your symptoms? Are you worried about anything in particular?"

Patient: *"I have had a bit of a look on Google but just came across so many different things – it was a bit baffling, to be honest. At the moment, I'm a bit frustrated at my lack of sleep but my GP has given me some sleeping tablets. They've helped a bit. I suppose my main concern is the impact any hand problem might have on my golf. I've played three or four times a week for the past thirty years and have made some great friends at the club. I wouldn't want to give it up. If I'm being honest with you, I am also a bit worried about what might be causing the problems with my hand. A good family friend was recently diagnosed with Parkinson's disease, and he first went to the doctor after he had some problems with clumsiness, doing up buttons, that kind of thing. I don't know if there's something sinister underlying all of this."*

What else would you like to ask?

You now have a clear picture of the nature and history of the presenting complaint and the patient's ideas, concerns and expectations. Complete your history by elucidating Mr. Wolfson's past medical and surgical history, drug history, social history and by conducting a brief systems review.

You: "Do you have any other health problems? Have you ever had surgery?"

Patient: *"Yes, now you mention it. I've had angina for the past four or five years, but it doesn't really stop me from walking round the golf course of taking the dogs out. I use my tongue spray if my chest does feel tight and that does the trick. I'm also diabetic – I was diagnosed about 10 years ago – and take metformin and gliclazide for that. I had a knee replacement three years ago, and (touchwood!) haven't had any problems since."*

You: "You've already mentioned your 'tongue spray', metformin & gliclazide. Do you take any other prescription medications? Anything over the counter?"

❝ **Patient:** *"Yes, I also take a statin for my cholesterol and amlodipine for my blood pressure. I also take cod liver oil tablets from my local chemist. I've tried some paracetamol for the tingling but it hasn't helped at all."*

You: "Can you tell me a bit about your home situation? Do you work?"

❝ **Patient:** *"I retired last year after working as a geography teacher at the local high school for thirty-two years. It's been great fun since – lots of golf, a few nice holidays and seeing plenty of the grandchildren. I live with my wife, Sarah. She's 63 and still working with the Council."*

How would you close the scenario?

If you feel you have obtained all relevant information from Mr. Wolfson, you can take the opportunity to summarise the history and repeat it back to the patient to demonstrate your attentive listening and to build rapport.

You: "So Mr. Wolfson, for the past three months, you've been experiencing a 'frustrating' tingling in your right hand, particularly at night. It affects your thumb, index finger and middle finger, but not your ring finger or pinky. You've also noticed that you've been more clumsy recently, but haven't had any thumb weakness affecting your writing or ability to grip objects. You're concerned about your disturbed sleep, any impact a hand problem might have on your golf, and a possible 'sinister' underlying cause. You also have angina, diabetes and had a successful right knee replacement three years ago. Have I missed anything out? Is there anything else that you'd like to add?"

❝ **Patient:** *"No, that's everything doctor. Well remembered!"*

What is your differential diagnosis?

Collectively, paresthesia within the distribution of the right median nerve, associated clumsiness, and the absence of weakness in thumb movements, are strongly suggestive of carpal tunnel syndrome. Other diagnoses to exclude are:
• Mononeuritis multiplex – diabetic peripheral neuropathy.
• Pronator teres syndrome.
• Anterior interosseous nerve syndrome.
• Degenerative arthritis at the hand and wrist.

Please explain your working diagnosis and management plan to the patient.

The patient has already voiced concerns about a possible 'sinister' underlying cause and it may therefore be helpful to provide appropriate reassurance at this point, particularly with respect to Parkinson's disease. Be clear in your explanation of what is causing the problem and treatment options.

You: "Mr. Wolfson, thank you for talking to me today and for allowing me to examine you. Several things might explain the tingling in your right hand and the increasing clumsiness you describe. Given your symptoms, some of the other things you've described, and my

HISTORIES

examination findings, I suspect that you have something called carpal tunnel syndrome. Have you heard this term before?"

66 **Patient:** *'No, doctor, I haven't heard of it.'*

You: "Well, many of the tendons, nerves and blood vessels that serve your hands run through a narrow space in the wrist called the carpal tunnel. One of these structures is the median nerve, which relays sensation from the thumb, index finger and middle finger and also controls some of your thumb movements. In carpal tunnel syndrome, this nerve becomes compressed, leading to tingling in those fingers and increased clumsiness. This closely matches your symptoms. You mentioned that you've had concerns about a sinister underlying cause of these symptoms. Carpal tunnel syndrome is very common and in most cases arises spontaneously in unlucky people due to their natural wrist anatomy. However, a subset of patients do have an underlying health problem such as an underactive thyroid gland. I don't suspect any underlying problem but we can run some blood tests to be sure. Would you like to discuss our treatment options?"

66 **Patient:** *'Yes please doctor.'*

You: "Well, first of all, we can offer you a wrist splint to hold your hand in a good position at night. This prevents the nerve from being compressed and so really helps with the night-time tingling and your quality of sleep. However, the splint would only control your symptoms, rather than solving the problem itself. We could also perform a short operation in which we release the pressure on the nerve, which should put a stop to the tingling and prevent the problem from progressing further. It's a very simple and effective procedure and most patients are usually in and out of hospital in a day. You may need to be admitted the night before due to your diabetes, but we can discuss this nearer the time if you decide to go through with the operation."

SUMMARY

Given this patient's past history of type II diabetes mellitus, use a structured history and focused questions to differentiate between carpal tunnel syndrome and mononeuritis multiplex. Focus on the functional impairment associated with the problem, notably the potential impact on the patient's ability to play golf and thus his social life.

Although this scenario appears quite straight forward do not forget communications skills principles. Check the patient's ideas, concerns and expectations. A family friend was recently diagnosed with Parkinson's disease which is particularly worrying the patient.

HISTORIES

🙂 Actor Brief

You are Brian Wolfson, a 66-year-old gentleman who has been experiencing a frustrating 'tingling' sensation in his right hand over the past three months. You are a recently retired secondary school teacher and live with your 63-year-old wife, Sarah, and your two dogs.

Presenting Complaint: The 'tingling' sensation only affects your right thumb, index finger, and middle finger, and feels like 'pins and needles', similar to when you 'bang your funny bone.' This sensation is worst at night and is severely disrupting your sleep. You've also noticed that you have been increasingly clumsy around the house, dropping mugs and knocking over other objects.

ICE: You are a keen golfer and fear that a hand problem could prevent you from playing as regularly as you would like to at your local club. Deep down, you're also concerned that these new symptoms may signal a more sinister underlying disease. A family friend was recently diagnosed with Parkinson's disease and he first went to a doctor as his tremor caused him to drop things.

PMH/SH: For the past four years, you have suffered with angina. However, you feel this is well controlled with your (GTN) tongue spray and has little, if any, impact on your ability to walk the dogs and play golf. You also take a statin and amlodipine to help your heart and blood pressure. You were diagnosed with type II diabetes nine years ago, which is managed with metformin and gliclazide. You have undergone surgery in the past – a successful total knee replacement aged 63.

TOP TIPS

➕ Use focused questions to glean necessary information from this reticent patient.

➕ Avoid jargon and be clear in your explanation of carpal tunnel syndrome, providing appropriate reassurance about underlying causes.

HISTORIES

3.7 | Calf Pain

Scenario

Your next patient in the vascular clinic is John Thompson, a gentleman aged 61 with a 1 week history of calf pain in his right leg.
You have washed your hands and introduced yourself, please take a history and suggest a management plan.

How would you begin?

Calf pain in a vascular clinic is indicative of a certain pathology, however it is important not to let presumptions dictate the opening of a history. Begin with an open question to provide you with more specific clues as to what Mr. Thompson is complaining of. Be sure not to interrupt too early with leading questions - you might miss key clues that way!

You: "Mr. Thompson, can you tell me about the problems you're having?"

66 **Patient:** *"For a few days now I have been getting sharp, stabbing pains in my right calf when I've been walking for a few minutes - makes me stop it does. But yesterday night I got the pain when I was watching TV, but worse. I can't be getting these pains, my wife is in a wheelchair and she relies on me to get her around!"*

What would you ask next?

Acknowledge that you understand the difficulties he must be going through. You need to find out more about the pain, however first discover whether he has any other symptoms to report. Remember, the symptoms that the patient reports without prompting are often those that cause them the most distress. If there are any concealed symptoms they may either be less important to the patient or the patient may be embarrassed about them. As always, you open, non-leading questions.

You: "That sounds like it must be very difficult for you, and therefore it's important that we find out why you are getting these pains. Can you tell me about any other symptoms you've been experiencing?"

66 **Patient:** *"My foot is a bit cold, definitely colder than the other one! I'm also struggling to walk because of a painful sore on my right heel - I thought that was just a blister but it's not healed in weeks. Aside from that I am fit as a fiddle - haven't been to the doctor in years!"*

What would you ask next?

The patient is demonstrating his stoic demeanor, and it seems this is all the information he is willing to donate to you without further prompts. Asking about his ideas, concerns and expectations is useful at this point, as it is gives clues as to how severe the patient thinks his symptoms are, and helps you understand whether his worries extend beyond his medical problems.

You: "What do you think is going on? What is your main concern? What were you expecting when you came here today?"

> **Patient:** *"At first I thought it was bad cramp, or a torn muscle - but then it happened when I wasn't using my legs yesterday so now I don't know. You'll be able to give me some pills to help and then I'll be on my way, right? I need to get back to helping my wife - she's housebound if I'm not there for her."*

What questions would you ask that would lead to a diagnosis?

Now that you have let the patient talk, you have developed a rapport with him so he feels comfortable to answer your next set of closed, focussed questions. Your questions should be used to try and rule out (or in) your differential diagnoses.

✏️ Focussed Calf Pain Questions

• Use the SOCRATES model to gain information about the pain in both his calf and his heel. Be sure to obtain an accurate time line.
• Focus on exacerbating and relieving factors, if he doesn't offer you any, specifically ask about whether elevation relieves or worsens the pain. Find out which problem stops his walking, the calf pain or the heel pain.
• Find out whether any trauma precipitated the pain or the heel "sore".
• Ask about associated symptoms, specifically: Angina, shortness of breath, impotence, cold feet, varicose veins, leg swelling, loss of sensation. (You need to find out what is the likely cause of what sounds like an ulcer on his heel).

> **Patient:** *"Three days ago, in the morning when I was walking to the shops I felt it, after about 100m it came on suddenly, like someone stabbed me in the leg. I had to stop and sit down for 10 minutes before I was able to get up again. Happened a couple of times the next day too. But yesterday, I had my feet up watching TV and it was agony. Same again when I got into bed - I found myself sleeping with my legs dangling off the side of the bed. The sore on my heel got very painful when I had my feet up too, but that's strange because it's just a blister isn't it, doc? And like I said my foot has been cold. No trauma though, nor varicose veins, or swelling. Come to mention it, I haven't had an erection for a while."*

What else would you like to ask?

You now have a clear picture of the presenting complaint and hopefully some differential diagnoses (If certain aspects of the history of presenting complaint aren't clear, ask further focused questions to obtain accurate information). Complete your history, by covering PMH, FH, DH, SH and systems review. Within each of the categories, ask about the risk factors for peripheral vascular disease.

You: "Do you have any other medical conditions?" (blood pressure, MI, diabetes)

> **Patient:** *"No! As I said, I'm fit as a fiddle."*

You: "Any illnesses in the family?"

> **Patient:** *"Dad died of a heart attack at 60, Mum lived 'til she was 85."*

HISTORIES

You: "Do you take any medications?"

66 **Patient:** *"They make me take a statin, but I don't know why - they give them to everyone my age though don't they?"*

(NB, it's important to ask these questions, even if the patient has declared their health as, in the case here, patient's may not understand their diseases or medications. Explain to the patient why he may be taking the statin)

You: "Do you smoke/drink?"

66 **Patient:** *"Nothing excessive - I smoke about 10 a day, and drink a couple of pints a night!"*

You: "You mentioned that you look after your wife, is it just the two of you at home? Are you working? Does anyone help you look after her?"
Tip - the questions have been listed here, but in reality you should ask them individually and listen to the answer rather than bombarding the patient with a string of questions.

66 **Patient:** *"I stopped working a few years ago to look after her, her sister comes and helps with the washing and the ironing a couple of times a week, but it's mostly just me and her. I was a builder."*

How would you close the scenario?

If you feel you have obtained all the necessary information you can from the patient, recount it back to him to help clarify the history in your head as well as giving him chance to interrupt if you have misunderstood certain statements.

You: "You started getting sudden stabbing pains in your right calf on walking to the shops 3 days ago, which was relieved by sitting down and resting for 10 minutes or so. Yesterday your got the same pain which wasn't precipitated by exercising. Your right foot was very cold too. You found the pain worse when you had your foot up, and it got better when you dangled your right leg off the edge of the bed. You also mention a painful sore on the right heel, which is similarly improved by lowering your feet. You take a statin, but are otherwise fit and well, and you are keen to get back home to support your wife who relies on your care. Have I missed anything?"

66 **Patient:** *"No, that's spot on, doc."*

Please explain your management plan to the patient

Be clear in your explanation to the patient about what you think he is describing and outline the care he will receive.

You: "The symptoms you are describing, and what I have seen on examination, point towards a problem within the blood vessels supplying your legs wherein they are narrowing. When you go walking, your legs need more oxygen for exercise, and the narrowing vessels can't supply all the oxygen your muscles need: this is why you were getting pain when you were walking to the shops. The sore on your heel is an ulcer, and is most probably caused by the same problem. It is important that we assess and treat you quickly, because if your vessels get any narrower, the blood supply can be entirely cut off. You will need to be admitted to hospital today so we can do some tests, and we may have to do an operation to widen the narrowed vessel in your leg using a small balloon. Clearly this is a lot to take in and you were not expecting that. Do you have any questions or is there anything you'd like me to go over again?"

6 6 **Patient:** *"No, that is all clear."*

SUMMARY

Be clear on the way to differentiate between the characteristic histories of patients' with arterial and venous disease. Listen out for key clues in the history to guide your differential diagnosis: In this case, the pain being worsened by elevation was a giveaway. However, always be suspicious, as the patient may have both arterial and venous pathology. You should also know the differences in appearances of arterial, venous and neuropathic ulcers.

Have a clear system in your head for history taking, and stick to it. In this case, the patient tried to convince you he has no medical problems, however, your drug history gave you clues as to his raised cholesterol which he wasn't aware of.

😐 Actor Brief

You are John Thompson, a 61-year-old male who is stoic and adamant about his reluctance to come to the doctor. However, you are keen for a quick fix to your leg pain which is stopping you from doing your daily activities. You are now a retired builder, and care for your wife who is disabled.

Presenting complaint: 3 day history of stabbing pain in your right calf precipitated by walking 100m. You got the pain at rest yesterday, and it is worsened by elevating your feet. You have an ulcer on your right heel, which has had a similar pain profile.

ICE: You think that the ulcer might be a blister, and the leg pain must be something to do with getting older. You want a tablet to make to help your symptoms so you can get back to looking after your wife.

PMH/DH/FH/SH: You smoke 10 cigarettes a day, drink 2 pints every night, and take a statin but you don't know why (you think they give them to all people who are "getting on a bit". Father died of a heart attack at 60.

TOP TIPS

➕ Win the patient's respect by listening and empathising with his social situation.

➕ Be clear and confident in your management plan. The patient was not expecting to be admitted and require an operation, so you will need to be ready to justify why he needs the proposed course of treatment.

HISTORIES

3.8   Dyspepsia

Scenario

Your next patient in the upper GI clinic is Richard Jones, a 52-year-old gentleman with a six week history of indigestion.

How would you begin?

Begin your consultation with an open question. It is important to let your patient speak without interruption as this will help to build the rapport between you and your patient. Allowing Mr. Jones to explain his symptoms may provide you with some clues as to the underlying pathology.

You: "Mr. Jones, can you tell me about the problems you're having?"

66 **Patient:** *"Well doctor, I've been getting this terrible indigestion. It started about a month and a half ago. Back then it was pretty mild, but recently it seems to be getting worse. In fact, it's really put me off my food and has made me pretty miserable!"*

What would you ask next?

First, you should empathise with the patient. At this early stage of the consultation it is important to find out if he has any other symptoms.
You: "I'm sorry to hear that Mr. Jones, it sounds like it's been giving you a lot of bother. Before we talk more about the indigestion, can you tell me if you've had any other symptoms?"

66 **Patient:** *"I think it might be because I'm not eating as much but I reckon I've lost some weight. I've not weighed myself so I don't know how much I've lost. My clothes seem a lot looser on me and I've had to use a tighter notch on my belt. My wife thinks that my face looks a lot thinner as well. Aside from that, I feel fine. I tend to get some back pain now and again but it doesn't bother me that much."*

What would you ask next?

Now you should focus on the presenting complaint. It is important to make sure you clarify the onset and progression of the symptoms and what the patient means by terms like "indigestion." If he is in any pain - it would be useful to use a framework like SOCRATES to assess it.

66 **Patient:** *"I remember the first time I got the indigestion, I had just had this spicy curry. At the time I thought I might have just had too much to eat. What do I mean by indigestion? Well I seem to get it just after I eat - I start off feeling really full. Then, I get this burning pain right in my chest. It's right in the middle of my chest and sometimes it moves upwards. It tends to last for 10-15 minutes and then goes*

away. I'm not sure if anything makes it better or worse but I really only notice it after I eat. I'd say it's about a 6/10 pain but to begin with it was only a 4."

What would you ask next?

Try and summarise what the patient has told you so far. Due to the anorexia, weight loss and progressive nature of the symptoms, this is beginning to resemble a worrying clinical picture. Now ask more focussed questions about the rest of his GI health.

✎ Focussed Dyspepsia Questions

• Associated GI symptoms: oral problems, dysphagia, nausea and vomiting, abdominal pain, change in bowel habit
• In dyspepsia histories remember to use the acronym ALARMS for red flag symptoms. **A**naemia, **L**oss of weight, **A**norexia, **R**ecent onset/progressive symptoms, **M**elaena/haematemesis, **S**wallowing difficulty.

❝❝ **Patient:** *"No I haven't felt particularly tired recently and I've always kept fit so I've not really noticed being out of breath. I think my chewing and swallowing have been fine - I've not had any problems with that and I've not felt nauseated or vomited since this indigestion started. I haven't had any tummy pains and my bowel movements are regular. I've not noticed any change in my stools either."*

What would you ask next?

Asking about the patient's ideas, concerns and expectations will help build your rapport with him and will allow you to pick up more information.

You: "What do you think is going on? What is your main concern? What were you expecting when you came here today?"

❝❝ **Patient:** *"At first, I thought I'd had a particularly spicy curry that didn't agree with me. However because it's been going on for so long, I think there might be something wrong with me. I'm worried that it's getting worse and that it's stopping me eating my meals. I just want to get the bottom of it and find out why I'm getting this indigestion."*

What else would you like to ask?

You should now have a clear picture of the presenting complaint and hopefully some differential diagnoses. If certain aspects of the history of presenting complaint are not clear, ask further focussed questions to obtain accurate information. Complete your history by covering PMH, DH, FH, SH and systems review. Within each section of the history, ask specifically about risk factors for Upper GI disease.
You: "Do you have any other medical conditions?" (Any other GI diseases, dietary changes)

❝❝ **Patient:** *"Just the back pain. I've had that for two years, I slipped on some ice a few winters ago."*

You: "Do you take any medications?" (NSAIDs, steroids, antibiotics)

> **Patient:** *"I take ibuprofen for my back. I've been taking it pretty regularly for about a year. It definitely helps with the pain."*

You: "Do you have any allergies?"

> **Patient:** *"No."*

You: "Anything that runs in the family?" (Peptic ulcer disease, cancer)

> **Patient:** *"Don't think so."*

You: "Do you smoke/drink?"

> **Patient:** *"I've smoked a pack a day for 25 years. I drink a couple of pints of Guinness every night."*

You: "What do you do for work? Who's at home with you?"
I'm a plasterer, these problems haven't really affected my work. I live with my wife and two sons.

How would you close the scenario?

To finish the history, summarise back what the patient has told you. A short summary will show the patient that you have been actively listening. It will also give him chance to clarify any misunderstandings.

You: "For the past month and a half, you've been getting this indigestion which has been steadily getting worse. You tend to feel fuller than usual after a meal and then you get a sense of heartburn. Due to the indigestion, you've lost your appetite and are not eating as much as you normally do. You also think you may have lost some weight. You take some ibuprofen for your back pain but are otherwise fit and well. Have I missed anything?"

> **Patient:** *"No that's everything doctor."*

SUMMARY

Due to presence of the ALARMS symptoms, this should be treated as a suspected gastric malignancy. Therefore an Upper GI endoscopy should be performed. If a mass or ulcer is found, then biopsies should be taken and analysed. Other investigations may be appropriate such as FBC - check for anaemia, ECG - rule out cardiac problem.

HISTORIES

☺ Actor Brief

You are Richard Jones, a 52 year old gentleman who is quite worried about his indigestion.

Presenting Complaint: 6 week history of indigestion. The indigestion comes on after eating. You feel fuller than you would normally expect and you get a burning pain in the middle of your chest. Due to this indigestion you have lost your appetite and feel like you're losing weight.

ICE: You thought the indigestion was due to eating a particularly spicy curry but because it has gone on for so long - you are starting to get worried. You just want to get to the bottom of your problems and find out the cause.

PMH/DH/FH/SH: You have had back pain for two years and take ibuprofen for it. You smoke a pack a day and drink a couple of pints of Guinness a night. You live with your wife and two sons.

TOP TIPS

✚ Remember the ALARMS acronym for patients with dyspepsia

✚ Use your communication skills and empathy to put the patient at ease and find out his ICE

✚ Remember to ask about other risk factors throughout the history. In this example - the patient's NSAID use and his smoking and drinking habits.

HISTORIES

3.9   Knee Injury

Scenario

You are the orthopaedic registrar on call. You have been asked to attend the Emergency Department to see Jessica Jones, a 27-year-old woman who twisted her left leg skiing in France 2 days ago. She was unable to continue and decided to catch the next plane back to the UK. Her leg has been giving way ever since. You have washed your hands and introduced yourself. Please take a history and suggest a management plan.

How would you begin?

Introduce yourself and check you have the right patient.

You: "Hello, I'm Dr. X and I'm the surgical SHO. May I just check, are you Jessica Jones?"

Begin with an open question and allow the patient to explain as much as she feels able to. A friendly facial expression, tone of voice, and body language are all much more important than the semantics of the words you use. Allow the patient to speak uninterrupted and use active listening whilst they give you the history.

You: "Can you tell me what has brought you in today?"

❝ **Patient:** *"I was skiing in France a couple of days ago and got knocked over by a bloody snowboarder! It was extremely painful, I had to get the ski-lift back down the mountain. It's just been so painful so I got the next plane home and came here."*

What would you ask next?

You should continue to gather information. Continue with open questions as these give the patient maximal opportunity to give you their history. Using closed questions too early on may ruin the patient's train of thought and you may miss something important.

Tip - The patient has told you that she was knocked over. If you use her own words in the opening of your question you will demonstrate that you were actively listening to her.

You: "You said you were knocked over...can you tell me more about exactly what happened/can you tell me more about how you fell?"

❝ **Patient:** *"It's hard to explain, my left ski got caught and I don't know, my left leg just kind of twisted under me as I fell."*

You: "You said it was extremely painful, I'm not surprised you couldn't ski on. Apart from the pain, did you notice anything else?"

Tip: This little phrase 'I'm not surprised you couldn't ski on' shows you are empathising with her and continues to build rapport.

66 **Patient:** *"Well, I felt it pop as I went down. When I got back down and took my gear off my knee was really swollen."*

What questions might point to a diagnosis?

Ask more focused questions to get to a diagnosis.

> ✎ **Comm Skills Tip: Signposting**
>
> **Tip:** Asking the patient's permission to focus on the main symptom signposts them to the fact that you are moving from open to more direct questioning. It is also a slick way of keeping the patient focused on the symptom and the question you asked and less likely to go off topic.

You: "Do you mind if I ask some specific questions about the knee?"

66 **Patient:** *"Yes please do."*

Ask about instability in the joint. This may give clues as to what structures are injured:
You: "Does the leg give way or has it ever locked?"

66 **Patient:** *"Yes actually, it keeps giving way, especially when walking downstairs. I can walk on it, but if I just twist on it ever so slightly it's excruciating."*

You: "And how about locking? Can you full bend and straighten it?"

True locking is the inability to completely flex or completely extend the joint.

66 **Patient:** *"Sort of. I can only bend it so far and then it just won't go any further."*

What else would you want to ask?

Ask about past medical history, relevant social history, medications and allergies etc. Also, use this opportunity to find out about the patient's ideas, concerns and expectations.

You: "Do you have any other medical problems?"

66 **Patient:** *"No, none."*

You: "Do you take any regular medications?"

66 **Patient:** *"Only my contraceptive pill."*

You: "Do you have any allergies?"

66 **Patient:** *"No."*

You: "Do you smoke or drink?"

HISTORIES

66 Patient: *"I don't smoke, I do like a drink on the weekends though, maybe 6 or 7 pints of cider."*

You: "What do you do for work?"

66 Patient: *"I'm an aerospace engineer."*

Ideas, concerns, and expectations

In any scenario the diagnoses may seem obvious to you but the patient may not be following your thought process and you need to elicit what they think this is. For example if a patient has a persistent cough and the history leads you to think it may be lung cancer, but you find out the patient just thinks it a simple viral infection, then you need to find this out early as it changes how you shape the rest of the consultation.

You: "Do you know what you might have done?"

66 Patient: *"Well I think I might have torn something but I'm praying I haven't."*

Even for the exact same injury, a patient's concerns will vary depending on their personal circumstances. You may think the patient's main concern should be how they will work or drive, but their biggest concern may be who will look after the cat whilst they're in hospital. Make no assumptions and treat all concerns seriously as they are issues about which the patient cares deeply.

You: "These injuries can create a lot of concern. Can you tell me about anything in particular that is worrying you?"

66 Patient: *"I'm worried how badly damaged it is, I go skiing 3 or 4 times a year, I don't know what I'll do if I can't ski again."*

With expectations, again you may feel the answer is obvious. But if the patient is terrified of surgery then you should have identified this before launching into the pros and cons of operative management and then detailing the post-operative rehabilitation regimen. Given that we don't have a definite diagnosis, rather than asking about expectations it might be better at this stage to focus on what will happen next.

You: "Do you know what's going to happen now?"

66 Patient: *"Well I expect I need some sort of a scan and then you'll tell me what's going to happen next. God I hope it's not something that needs an operation!"*

How would you close the consultation?

Now that you have come to the end of your history it is good practise to summarise back to the patient to ensure you have all the facts. This also allows her the opportunity to add/correct anything. After summarising you can check there is nothing else she wishes to add before thanking her and explaining what your management plan is.

You: "OK, just to check I haven't missed anything can I just clarify what you've told me"

66 Patient: *"Of course."*

HISTORIES

You: 'So you fell two days ago, your left leg twisted underneath you, you felt it pop and it swelled up very quickly. It's been very painful since, especially if you twist it. The knee also feels unstable and gives way, more so walking downstairs, and you're not able to bend it as far as normally. Is there anything else you'd like me to know?"

66 **Patient:** *"No I think that's everything."*

Please explain your management plan to the patient?

It is important to explain your diagnosis clearly to the patient and how you would manage this, giving them the opportunity to ask questions.
Tip - it is a nice touch to signpost the explanation and say that you are happy for questions.

You: "I'm going to explain what's going to happen next. Please stop me if you'd like me to clarify anything or go over anything again.
It sounds like you may have injured some of the ligaments and cartilage in your knee. The first step is to make sure we get your pain under control and stop any further damage from occurring so we will make sure you have enough painkillers and we need to put your leg into a splint to keep the knee immobile. We'll get you an X-ray to check the bones and make sure there are no fractures but we will also need to get an MRI of your knee to fully assess the ligaments and the cartilage. This can be done as an outpatient. If the MRI shows us there is damage to the soft tissue inside the knee, it's very likely that you will need surgery to reconstruct the ligaments and cartilage. Is there anything you'd like to ask me?"

66 **Patient:** *"If I have surgery, how long am I likely to be out of action?"*

You: "ACL ruptures in a young, active patient like yourself will almost always need to be surgically reconstructed in order to stabilise the knee.
A graft ligament will be taken from near the knee, either the patella or hamstring tendon, and fixed into the knee using keyhole surgery techniques. The damaged meniscus can be assessed at the same time and either repaired or trimmed as necessary.
If we repair the meniscus with a stitch we will ask you to mobilise touch weight-bearing with crutches for 6 weeks before fully weight-bearing. If we trim the meniscus you can weight-bear full straight away which is what we routinely do for the ACL reconstruction. You will have physio straight away and we will restrict the amount of bend in you knee for the first few months to protect the graft.
She should be able to return to her normal level of activity after around 6 weeks and get back to sports at around 6 months."

66 **Patient:** *"OK, thank you for explaining things to me."*

SUMMARY

The mechanism of injury in this case, twisting of the knee with the foot planted, is typical for anterior cruciate ligament tear, one of the most common knee injuries. It is often sustained playing football, rugby, or skiing.
ACL injuries are more common in women, and can often occur in conjunction with damage to other soft tissue structures in the knee, such as the PCL, the menisci, or the collaterals. Your history should focus on trying to tease out which of these structures may be involved. Surgical reconstruction is almost always required to regain normal function.

HISTORIES

🙂 Actor Brief

You are Jessica Jones, a 27-year-old aerospace engineer. Two days ago you were skiing in Val d'Isère when you were clipped by snowboarder and fell. It was extremely painful and you had to take the ski lift back down the mountain and got the first plane home.

Presenting complaint: Your left ski was stuck in the snow, so as you fell your knee twisted underneath you and you felt it pop. When you took your gear off later, you noticed it had swollen considerably. The pain is inside the knee joint itself, about 4-5/10 but if you twist it, it feels like a hot knife and goes to 9/10. It's not too bad if you don't move the knee. When questioned further, you confess that while you are able to put weight on it, it gives way, more so walking down hill or down stairs. You can bend the knee but not as far as normally, it feels stuck and is more painful.

ICE: You are an avid skier and are really worried you've done irreparable damage to your knee that will prevent you from skiing again. When the doctor mentions surgery, all you really want to know is how long the recovery period will be.

PMH/DH/SH: You are normally fit & well, the only medication you take regularly is your contraceptive pill and you have no allergies. You don't smoke, and you drink 6-7 pints of cider a week, usually just at weekends.

TOP TIPS

➕ Remember to consider the possibility that there may be more than one pathology.

➕ Asking thorough questions about instability and locking can help you work out the diagnosis.

➕ Show empathy. Skiing is a big part of the patient's life and she is scared she may not be able to do it again. Never trivialise any of the patient's concerns.

3.10 | Urinary Retention

> ## Scenario
>
> Your next patient on the surgical assessment unit is Francis Underwood, a 70-year-old man who has been referred in from the Emergency Department with acute urinary retention. The nurse has scanned his bladder, revealing a residual volume of 1500mLs. He has been catheterised and over 1L drained and is now much more comfortable.
>
> You have washed your hands and introduced yourself. Please take a history and suggest a management plan.

How would you begin?

Start with an open question and find out why the patient has come in.

You: "Can you tell me what it is that has brought you in?"

❝ **Patient:** *"Well I'm not really sure. I've not been able to pass water for the last two days and it's become very painful"*

What would you ask next?

Continue with open-ended questions to gather more information, and avoid closed questions at this early stage of the consultation.

You: "Can you tell me more?"

❝ **Patient:** *"Well it's basically that. What else would you like to know?"*

Tip - if despite open questioning the patient gives you very short answers or may not understand what you want to know, then you may start using more focused question to start to explore the presenting symptom and ask about any associated symptoms.

You: "Have you noticed anything else?'

❝ **Patient:** *"Not really."*

You: "Have you noticed any other troubling symptoms?"

❝ **Patient:** *"The urination has been playing up for a few months though."*

You: "Can you tell me what you mean?"

❝ **Patient:** *"It's just been getting quite difficult to go recently."*

What questions might point to a diagnosis?

Ask more focused closed, urological questions to reach a diagnosis:

HISTORIES

> 🖉 **Focussed Urinary Retention Questions**
>
> • How long has the difficulty been for?
> • Difficulty initiating?
> • 'Stopping' and 'starting'?
> • Any dysuria?
> • Increased frequency?
> • Does he experience any post-void dribbling?
> • Any episodes of incontinence?
> • Sensation of incomplete voiding?
> • Nocturia?
> • Haematuria?

66   **Patient:** *"I couldn't tell you exactly when it started, but it's been a few months. It's quite difficult to get started, and then it's only a dribble. It's not painful, but it feels like I still need to go, even after I've gone! I do sometimes get some dribbling afterwards but no actual accidents. I'm peeing about 8 or 9 times a day and have to get up 2 or 3 times in the night to go. I haven't noticed any blood in the water though."*

Remember to ask about red flag symptoms:

• Pelvic pain?
• Back pain?
• Any bowel troubles/incontinence?
• Any weight loss?

66   **Patient:** *"I've not had any pain no, I'm still very active and don't really get back pain. Bowels are absolutely fine, although I do get a bit constipated sometimes, and my weight has been stable."*

What else would you want to ask?

Ask about past medical history, relevant social history, medications and allergies etc. Also, use this opportunity to find out about the patient's ideas, concerns and expectations.

You: "Do you have any other medical problems?"

66   **Patient:** *"None at all, I'm in pretty good shape."*

You: "Do you take any regular medications?"

66   **Patient:** *"None."*

You: "Do you have any allergies?"

66   **Patient:** *"Just to latex."*

You: "Do you smoke/drink?"

66   **Patient:** *"Never smoked, I have a gin & tonic every night."*

HISTORIES

You: "Are you currently working?"

66 **Patient:** *"No, I used to be a banker, I retired about 5 years ago."*

You: "What do you think may be going on? Is there anything in particular you're worried about?"

66 **Patient:** *"I'm not really sure, I don't particularly want it to happen again though!"*

How would you close the consultation?

Summarise your history back; this demonstrates to the patient that you have paid attention to them and gives them the opportunity to add/correct anything. After summarising, check there is nothing else the patient wants to add before thanking them and explaining your management plan.

You: "You've been having difficulty passing water for a few months now, in that it's difficult to start, the stream is quite weak and you don't feel you've fully emptied your bladder. You are also going more often and getting up frequently in the night to go. Then you've not been able to go at all for the last two days. Is there anything else you'd like me to know?"

66 **Patient:** *"Yes, it was bloody painful when they put that catheter in!"*

Please explain your management plan to the patient

It is important to explain your diagnosis clearly to the patient and how you would manage this, giving them the opportunity to ask questions.

You: "From the history you've given me, I believe you have an enlargement of the prostate gland, which surrounds the tube that runs out of the bladder to urinate. The enlargement compresses the tube and can cause all the difficulties you've had passing water. As for what is causing the swelling, this can just occur naturally as we become older, it can be a result of infection or sometimes it can be due to cancer and this is something I think we need to rule out. I will need to perform an examination of the back passage to assess your prostate gland, we will take some blood tests to check your kidneys haven't been affected too badly and we will need to get a biopsy of the prostate. Is there anything you'd like to ask me?"

66 **Patient:** *"How is the biopsy done?"*

You: "An ultrasound probe is passed into the back passage and this is used to guide a small needle through the wall of the rectum into the prostate to take a tissue sample for testing. It can be uncomfortable so you will be given some local anaesthetic. There are some risks, such as minor bleeding and infection, and there is a possibility the biopsy may miss a cancer if it is not in the area of tissue sampled."

How would you manage benign prostatic hypertrophy in this patient?

• In the first incidence, lifestyle changes such as limiting caffeine and alcohol intake, and regular exercise may help mild symptoms.
• This may be tried in combination with medication such as 5α-reductase inhibitors (finasteride, dutasteride) and alpha blockers (tamsulosin).
• The patient may need to be discharged with a temporary catheter and followed up in a specialist nurse clinic.

HISTORIES

• If these interventions fail to relieve the symptoms, the patient may need consideration for surgery, such as transurethral resection of prostate (TURP).

SUMMARY

You should aim to take a thorough urological history and focus on red flag symptoms, as prostate cancer must be ruled out in an older male with urinary retention.
Benign prostatic hypertrophy/hyperplasia is relatively common in men over 50 and can lead to retention. BPH does NOT increase risk of developing prostate cancer.
Remember that a digital rectal examination can lead to falsely elevated PSA thus any blood tests should be taken PRIOR to examination.

😐 Actor Brief

You are Francis ("Frank") Underwood, a 70-year-old retired investment banker. You were brought into A&E in excruciating pain after not being able to urinate for the last two days. You feel much better after a catheter is inserted although the actual passing was very uncomfortable.

Presenting complaint: You haven't passed water for the last two days and it has been causing increasing pain in your abdomen. When the doctor asks if you have noticed anything else, you mention that you've been having issues with urination for a few months. When questioned further, you inform the doctor that you have difficulty initiating urination, the stream is quite poor, stops and starts, and you feel like you haven't fully emptied the bladder afterwards. You are going more often, up to 9 times a day, and getting up 2-3 times a night to pass water. You have not noticed any blood, and there is no pain passing water.

ICE: You aren't sure what is going on, all you know is that you don't want it to happen again. When the doctor mentions a biopsy, you want to know what this will involve.

PMH/DH/SH: You are very fit and active still, take no medication and are allergic to latex. You are a life-long non-smoker and have a small gin & tonic every night. You have no significant family history.

TOP TIPS

➕ Make sure you know the red flag symptoms of prostate malignancy

➕ Did you spot that the patient was allergic to latex? Some catheters are made of latex rubber or Teflon-coated latex- it is important to check what kind of catheter has been inserted!

➕ In this patient, who is not sure what may be the cause of his problems, and may potentially have a malignancy, it is essential to find a balance between informing him of what may be going on without being too alarmist.

3.11 | Abdominal Pain

Scenario

You are on the surgical assessment unit on Sunday evening; your next patient to see is Lana Kane, a 40-year-old woman. She has been admitted with abdominal pain and nausea. The pain has been constant for the last 12 hours and she can no longer tolerate it.

You have washed your hands and introduced yourself. Please take a history and suggest a management plan.

How would you begin?

Start with an open question and find out why the patient has come to ED.
You: "Can you tell me what has been happening?"

66 **Patient:** *"I've got this pain in my tummy, right at the top, it's just been getting worse all day and I'm in agony now."*

What would you ask next?

Use open-ended questions to gather more information, try to avoid closed questions at the beginning of the consultation. Explore the presenting symptom and ask about any associated symptoms.

You: "Apart from the pain, has there been anything else?"

66 **Patient:** *"I feel so sick as well, I tried to eat dinner this evening but it just made me feel worse"*

What questions might point to a diagnosis?

Ask more focused closed questions to reach a diagnosis

Focussed Abdominal Pain Questions

- Where exactly is the pain?
- What brings the pain on?
- What does it feel like?
- Does the pain move anywhere else?
- Does anything make the pain better/worse?
- How bad is the pain on a scale of 1-10?

66 **Patient:** *"It's all here (indicates epigastrium and right upper quadrant), it started this afternoon after Sunday lunch, it was just a twinge but it hasn't gone off since, its just getting worse gradually, it feels sharp. Nothing is helping the pain. It's about 9 out of 10 now."*

Ask more about the nausea:

HISTORIES

• Is it associated with the pain? Which was present first?
• Has she just felt sick or actually vomited?

> **Patient:** *"It came on after the pain, more so in the last couple of hours, after I tried to eat some toast this evening. I vomited twice in A&E."*

Enquire about the presence of other symptoms, specifically bowel & urinary symptoms;

> **Patient:** *"I haven't noticed anything different when I open my bowels, but my urine looked quite dark when I gave a sample. I think I must be dehydrated."*

What else would you want to ask?

Ask about past medical history, relevant social history, medications and allergies etc. Also, use this opportunity to find out about the patient's ideas, concerns and expectations.
You: "Do you have any other medical problems?"

> **Patient:** *"No."*

You: "Do you take any regular medications?"

> **Patient:** *"My GP put me on a statin last month."*

You: "Do you have any allergies?"

> **Patient:** *"Penicillin, it gives me really bad diarrhoea."*

You: "Do you smoke/drink?"

> **Patient:** *"I've cut down the cigarettes, I only smoke about 15 a day now. I get through maybe 8 or 9 bottles of wine a week with my partner."*

You: "What do you do for work?"

> **Patient:** *"I'm a full-time mum, I have a 6-year-old and a 3-year-old at home."*

You: "What do you think may be going on? Is there anything in particular you're worried about?"

> **Patient:** *"I have no idea, I just want to get rid of this pain, it's becoming unbearable."*

How would you close the consultation?

Summarise your history back; this demonstrates to the patient that you have paid attention to them and gives them the opportunity to add/correct anything. After summarising, check there is nothing else the patient wants to add before thanking them and explaining your management plan.

HISTORIES

You: 'So since this lunchtime today, you've had this pain at the top on the right, initially it wasn't too bad but it's been getting worse all day and now it's 9/10 and nothing is helping the pain. You've also felt sick this evening and have vomited twice. You also mentioned that your urine looked dark. Is there anything else you'd like me to know?'

66 **Patient:** *"It also really hurts if I take a deep breath."*

Please explain your management plan to the patient

It is important to explain your diagnosis clearly to the patient and how you would manage this, giving them the opportunity to ask questions

You: "From everything you've told me, it sounds very likely that you have cholecystitis, an infection of the gallbladder brought on by gallstones getting stuck. Firstly we will make sure we get your pain and sickness under control so we'll give you some painkillers and anti-sickness medication. We'll need to take some blood tests, this can tell us if your body is fighting an infection, if so we'll start you on some antibiotics. The blood tests can also tell us if your liver is being affected which might suggest gallstones, but the best way for us to see what is happening with the gallbladder is an ultrasound scan so we will arrange that test as well. If these investigations all point to gallstones, then you may need an operation to remove the gallbladder. Is there anything you'd like to ask?"

66 **Patient:** *"When would the operation be?"*

You: "Typically, if you symptoms occur within 24 hours we will try and perform a cholecystectomy during the same admission on an emergency list. If your symptoms have been present for longer than this, it may be preferable to treat the acute phase with antibiotics and consider elective cholecystectomy when the episode has resolved. I will discuss the case with the team and get back to you as to which is the better option in your case."

66 **Patient:** *"Thank you for the information, that has been very helpful."*

SUMMARY

Gallstones may be present asymptomatically in many people; they rarely become an issue until they block off the gallbladder leading to acute cholecystitis
Gallstones are more common in the overweight/obese, in women, especially those who have had children, and in people over 40.
Untreated, gallstones can lead to cholangitis, acute pancreatitis or gallstone ileus, all of which can be followed by significant morbidity.

> 😐 **Actor Brief**
>
> You are Lana Kane, a 40-year-old full time mum of two. You've come into hospital on a Sunday evening with pain in your stomach that's been getting worse since lunch time.

Presenting complaint: The pain started after Sunday lunch as a dull twinge but has progressively gotten worse through the day until it has now become unbearable. The pain is epigastric and right upper quadrant, now a 9/10. You've also felt sick this evening, which started after trying to eat some toast. You vomited twice in A&E. When questioned, you also mention that your urine looked very dark when you gave a sample, but you assume its because you're dehydrated. When the doctor clarifies your story, you also mention that the pain gets worse when you take a deep breath in.

ICE: You are not sure what is going on, you just want it sorted ASAP as you can no longer tolerate the pain. When the doctor mentions an operation, you want to know how soon this can be done.

PMH/DH/SH: You have no medical history, but you do take the statin your GP prescribed last month. You tell the doctor that you are allergic to penicillin, but only reveal that it just gives you diarrhoea if specifically asked about reaction. You smoke 15 cigarettes a day and share 8-9 bottles of wine a week with your partner.

TOP TIPS

➕ Did you notice that the patient's reaction to penicillin is a side effect; therefore it should be safe to treat her with penicillin based antibiotics

➕ The patient is becoming increasingly uncomfortable with the pain; remember that timely analgesia is essential.

➕ Lifestyle advice may also make up an important component of your management plan, advising the patient to eat a more balanced diet, exercise regularly and reduce her excessive alcohol intake.

HISTORIES

3.12 Dysphagia

Scenario

Ms. Mallory Archer, a 55-year-old accountant, has been referred to your ENT clinic by her GP. The GP letter states that she has been complaining of dysphagia and halitosis, which has gotten worse over the last few weeks.

You have washed your hands and introduced yourself. Please take a history and suggest a management plan.

How would you begin?

Start with an open question and find out why the patient has come to see you.
You: "Can you tell me what has been going on?"

66 **Patient:** *"Well I've been having difficulty swallowing over the last couple of weeks, I went to see my GP and she sent me here."*

What would you ask next?

Use open-ended questions to gather more information, try to avoid closed questions at the beginning of the consultation. Explore the presenting symptom and ask about any associated symptoms.
You: "Have you noticed any other symptoms?"

66 **Patient:** *"Well I sort of felt that my breath smelt a bit, then my young grandson told me my breath smells as well! I brush my teeth twice a day, but it makes no difference!"*

What questions might point to a diagnosis?

When you feel the patient has said all they want, ask more focused, closed questions to get to a diagnosis.

Explore the dysphagia symptoms:
• Is there difficulty swallowing solids/ liquids/ both?'
• Does she cough/choke on food?
• Does the food come back up? Is there regurgitation?

66 **Patient:** *"It's mainly solid food, I haven't had any problem with liquids. I've choked a couple of times, but that stopped when I cut my food into smaller pieces. I haven't had any food coming back up, it just feels like it gets stuck going down."*

When a patient presents with dysphagia, remember to ask about respiratory symptoms:
• Any shortness of breath?
• If so, when does it come on?

66 **Patient:** *"No, I get a bit out of breath if I do too much, but I've been like that for a couple of years."*

HISTORIES

Dysphagia can be a sign of malignancy, remember to ask about red flag symptoms:
• Any weight loss?
• Any change in voice / hoarseness?
• Any pain?

66   **Patient:** *"No, if anything I've actually put weight on! I haven't noticed any change in my voice. I've not had any pain."*

What else would you want to ask?

Ask about past medical history, relevant social history, medications and allergies etc. Also, use this opportunity to find out about the patient's ideas, concerns and expectations.

You: "Do you have any other medical problems?"

66   **Patient:** *"High blood pressure and angina, but they don't really trouble me. I was diagnosed with reflux disease about 6 months ago."*

You: "Do you take any regular medications?"

66   **Patient:** *"Ramipril, diltiazem and aspirin. I have a GTN spray but I don't need to use it very often."*

You: "Do you have any allergies?"

66   **Patient:** *"No."*

You: "Do you smoke/drink?"

66   **Patient:** *"I used to smoke 20 a day but I quit about 6 years ago. I don't really drink, maybe a glass or two of champagne on special occasions."*

You: "What do you think may be going on? Is there anything in particular you're worried about?"

66   **Patient:** *"I'm sure I'm just being silly, but I'm scared it might be cancer. Everything seems to cause cancer nowadays."*

You: "Your concern is certainly understandable. Given what you've told me, cancer is unlikely but it is something we will investigate thoroughly. Do you have any family history of cancers?"

66   **Patient:** *"My father had prostate cancer. He died of a heart attack though."*

How would you close the consultation?

Summarise your history back; this demonstrates to the patient that you have paid attention to them and gives them the opportunity to add/correct anything. After summarising, check there is nothing else the patient wants to add before thanking them and explaining your management plan.

You: "For the last couple of weeks you've been having difficulty swallowing solid food, occasionally coughing on it but cutting it into smaller bits helps, you have had no problems swallowing liquids and no issues with regurgitating food, no weight loss or breathing difficulties. You also commented on some bad breath. Is there anything else you'd like to add?"

66 **Patient:** *"No I think that covers everything."*

What is the differential diagnosis?

In this patient the history is more suggestive of a mechanical blockage, rather than a motility disorder, so my differentials would include:
• Oesophageal web/ring
• Pharyngeal pouch
• Malignancy should be considered with a history of dysphagia, although there are no other red flag symptoms in this case.

What investigations would aid your diagnosis?

Bloods: specifically FBC (check for anaemia), U&Es, LFTs (potentially deranged secondary to metastatic disease) and albumin.
Endoscopy is necessary to rule out oesophageal malignancy.
Given the possibility of a pharyngeal pouch, endoscopy can be dangerous due to risk of perforation and a barium swallow may be safer, but the need to rule out malignancy takes priority.
CT scan may be required to screen for an external mass compressing oesophagus if other tests are negative.

Please explain your management plan to the patient

It is important to explain your diagnosis clearly to the patient and how you would manage this, giving them the opportunity to ask questions

You: "It sounds most likely that you have a ring of soft tissue encroaching in your oesophagus causing a narrowing, or possibly a little 'pouch' that is catching food. However, I think it is important that we rule out a malignancy. We need to check your bloods to see if there any abnormalities that may point to a diagnosis, but the main investigation we need to organise is a camera test to look at the inside of the oesophagus and check to see what's causing the blockage. If this doesn't show anything then we may need to get a CT scan to see what else could be causing the problem. Is there anything you'd like to ask me?"

66 **Patient:** *"It is quite a bit to take in, but I think you have covered everything. Thank you."*

SUMMARY

Oesophageal webs are thin membranes of normal oesophageal mucosa and submucosa, which can protrude into and subsequently occlude the oesophagus. They are more common in women and are usually located in the upper or middle part of the oesophagus.
It is important to consider malignancy in this scenario and thus your history should focus on asking about red flag symptoms.
Both oesophageal webs and pharyngeal pouches can be perforated during endoscopy, however endoscopy is indicated by the presence of dysphagia in this 55-year-old patient.

HISTORIES

😐 Actor Brief

You are Mallory Archer, a 55-year-old accountant. You went to see your GP recently because you were finding it increasingly difficult to swallow and your GP referred you to the ENT clinic.

Presenting complaint: Over the last couple of weeks, you have found it increasingly difficult to swallow. You have also noted that your breath smells, despite good dental hygiene. Your 4-year-old grandson also commented on your bad breath. When quizzed, you reveal that the difficulty is only with solid foods, and has caused a couple of coughing fits. You cut your food up smaller now and the coughing has stopped but it still feels like food is getting stuck in your throat. You haven't had any problems with food coming back up. You have no breathing difficulties, no weight loss and no change in your voice.

ICE: Your main concern is that you may have cancer, however you feel you may be over-reacting. When asked about your family history you reveal that your father had prostate cancer, although it was a heart attack that led to his death. When the doctor mentions sending you for a camera test you want to know how soon this will be.

PMH/DH/SH: You have hypertension and angina for which you take ramipril, diltiazem, aspirin and a GTN spray although you do not need to use the spray very often. You were diagnosed with reflux disease 6 months ago (only reveal that you take no medication for this if specifically asked). You have no allergies. You are an ex-smoker, having quit your 20-a-day habit 6 years ago. You only drink on special occasions (a glass or two of champagne).

TOP TIPS

➕ Did you pick up on the fact that this patient has a diagnosis of GORD but is not on any medication for it? A regular PPI may help reduce her risk of future webs forming, as well as providing some relief from her reflux

➕ The patient mentions that she is concerned about cancer but admits she feels silly to worry about this, it is important to reassure her and make her feel that you are taking her concerns seriously and will investigate thoroughly

➕ A thorough history regarding the dysphagia will quickly help differentiate between a mechanical or a motility issue.

3.13 Swollen Arm

Scenario

Your next patient in fracture clinic is Walter White, a 58-year-old teacher who was injured in a road traffic collision 3 months ago. He sustained a right-sided clavicle fracture, which was treated conservatively. His physiotherapist who has noted his right arm becomes swollen and discoloured after therapy sessions has referred him back.

You have washed your hands and introduced yourself. Please take a history and suggest a management plan.

How would you begin?

Start with an open question and find out why the patient has come to see you.

You: "Hello, I'm Dr. X from the surgical team. Can you tell me what has been happening?"

66 **Patient:** *"I was in a car crash a few months ago and broke my collar bone. Since then, my whole arm has been getting quite painful and swollen."*

What would you ask next?

Use open-ended questions to gather more information, try to avoid closed questions at the beginning of the consultation. Explore the presenting symptom and ask about any associated symptoms.

You: "Have you noticed any other symptoms?"

66 **Patient:** *"Well it seems to go blue the more swollen it gets. I thought it was my imagination but then the physio commented on it as well."*

What questions might point to a diagnosis?

Ask more focused closed questions to get to a diagnosis.
First use SOCRATES to ascertain a history of any pain.

66 **Patient:** *"It's all down my right arm, and into my hand. It's not too bad in the morning but over the course of the day it gets worse, especially if I'm writing on the whiteboard a lot. It's like very bad pins and needles, about 7-8/10. Resting it seems to make it better."*

Explore the swelling and discolouration:
• When does it come on?
• Is it linked to the pain?
• What makes it better?

66 **Patient:** *"It gets more swollen throughout the day as it becomes more painful. Again, the more I use the arm, the worse it gets."*

HISTORIES

With a history of sensory deficit, remember to enquire about motor symptoms also:
• Any weakness?
• Where?
• Is it constant or intermittent?

66 **Patient:** *"Yes actually, by the last lesson of the day I really struggle to hold the whiteboard pen. My whole hand feels weak but particularly my little finger."*

What else would you want to ask?

Ask about past medical history, relevant social history, medications and allergies etc.
Also, use this opportunity to find out about the patient's ideas, concerns and expectations.

You: "Do you have any other medical problems?"

66 **Patient:** *"Just high blood pressure, but I take ramipril and it doesn't cause me any trouble."*

You: "Do you have any allergies?"

66 **Patient:** *"No."*

You: "Do you smoke/drink?"

66 **Patient:** *"I don't smoke, I drink maybe 3 or 4 glasses of wine a week."*

You: "What do you do for work?"

66 **Patient:** *"I teach chemistry in secondary school."*

You: "Is there anything in particular about this that is concerning you?"

66 **Patient:** *"Well, I just want it fixed really. My wife doesn't work, it's just me support-ing the family and I can't work like this, it's just getting worse and worse."*

How would you close the consultation?

Summarise your history back; this demonstrates to the patient that you have paid atten-tion to them and gives them the opportunity to add/correct anything. After summarising, check there is nothing else the patient wants to add before thanking them and explaining your management plan.
You: "Since your accident you have noticed progressive pain down the right arm and hand, like pins and needles which becomes worse at work as you're writing on the board and gets better with rest. The arm becomes swollen and blue as well and you have no-ticed weakness in the hand also. Is there anything else you think I may have missed?"

66 **Patient:** *"No, that's everything."*

What is the differential diagnosis?

Given the history of recent clavicle fracture, the most likely diagnosis should be thoracic outlet obstruction secondary to malunion.
Brachial plexus injury could also be considered, but this is less likely in the context of swelling and discolouration this suggests a vascular component.

After clinical examination, what investigations would aid your diagnosis?

Thoracic outlet syndrome is usually a clinical diagnosis based on history and examination findings (Adson's test can be used but has low sensitivity and specificity).
In this case, it is important to obtain an X-ray to assess the clavicle fracture for evidence of non-/malunion.
EMG to assess the function of the brachial plexus, which is at risk of injury.

Please communicate your management plan to the patient

It is important to explain your diagnosis clearly to the patient and how you would manage this, giving them the opportunity to ask questions.

You: "I think the most likely diagnosis is thoracic outlet syndrome; this is what happens when the nerves and vessels running underneath the collar bone become compressed. In your case, it's quite likely this is because the fracture isn't healing properly and is pressing on those nerves and vessels, which is what's causing your symptoms. We need to get an XR today to check the position of the fracture and to see how it is healing and I'd like to refer you for some tests that look at the electrical activity of the nerves in your arm and hand to check for any damage. Is there anything you'd like to ask me?"

66 **Patient:** *"If it is because the fracture isn't healing properly, what will you do?"*

How would you manage this patient's clavicle fracture?

It is important to explain the procedure you intend to do and the benefits and risks of the operation.
You: "We will make a cut over the break, remove the callous that has formed, bring the two ends of the bone back together and fix a plate across the bone. The reason we want to do this is to treat the symptoms you are getting from the thoracic outlet syndrome. After this you will need some physiotherapy to ensure your shoulder range of movement returns quickly. The procedure has some risks, the main ones being having some irritation from the plate, developing a pneumothorax, the fracture still not healing correctly or us damaging your lung or blood vessels beneath the clavicle."

SUMMARY

Your history should pick up on the fact that this patient's symptoms are exacerbated by prolonged use of his right arm, i.e.- writing on a board at school. The swelling is a result of subclavian vein obstruction.
The recent clavicle fracture hints towards a malunion causing thoracic outlet obstruction.
Thoracic outlet obstruction is most often due to trauma or repetitive strain, but can also be caused by congenital abnormalities (cervical rib, anterior/middle scalene muscle abnormalities) or, rarely, tumours (i.e. Pancoast).

HISTORIES

☺ Actor Brief

You are Walter White, a 58-year-old chemistry teacher. You were in a car accident 3 months ago and broke your right collarbone.

Presenting complaint: For the last three months you have noticed progressively worsening pain and swelling spreading down your right arm, particularly at school when writing on the whiteboard. The pain is 7-8/10 and feels like intense pins and needles, especially in the little finger. When you are questioned further, you confess that it looks a little bluish too. You thought it was just your imagination but then the physiotherapist commented on it as well. The hand also feels weak by the end of the day, you struggle to hold a pen.

ICE: You are getting frustrated, as the pain and weakness is causing you great difficulty at work and you are worried you will not be able to continue teaching, as you are the sole earner in your household.

Significant PMH/DH/SH: You are normally fit and well, you only take ramipril for your high blood pressure. You have no allergies. You don't smoke, and you drink 3-4 glasses of wine a week. You live at home with your wife and son, and have a baby daughter on the way.

TOP TIPS

➕ Remember to take a thorough history of the neurology in the arm i.e. sensory/motor deficits. This will point to the lesion.

➕ Show empathy! This gentleman is concerned he will no longer be able to work due to his symptoms, and thus unable to support his family

➕ When going through consent for surgery, it is important to explain both general risks of surgery, and risks specific to the procedure being consented for, and allow the patient opportunity to ask questions/clarify anything they did not understand.

HISTORIES

3.14 | Hearing Loss

> ## Scenario
>
> Your next patient is Debbie Michaels, a 32-year-old lady. She has been referred by the GP to the ENT clinic with persistent ear discharge and a new change in hearing. You have washed your hands. Please take a history and suggest a management plan.

How would you begin?

Introduce yourself and check you have the right patient.
You: "Hello, I'm John Smith/Jane Smith and I'm the surgical SHO. May I just check, are you Debbie Michaels?"

Begin with an open question and allow the patient to explain as much as she feels able to. A friendly facial expression, tone of voice, and body language are all much more important than the semantics of the words you use. Allow the patient to speak uninterrupted and use active listening whilst they give you the history.

You: "Tell me what has brought you here today."

66 **Patient:** *"I've had horrible discharge from my right ear for about a year now. It's yellowy in colour and occasionally there are streaks of blood mixed in. It smells quite bad and I can't do anything to get rid of the odour. I've had every antibiotic and ear drop available but it always comes back. In the last month I think my hearing has got worse as well which is really worrying."*

Tip: If the patient is only giving small chunks of information at a time, then phrases such as "please go on" and "please tell me more" associated with an appropriate tone of voice and body language will invite them to tell you more. Remember, the more they tell you, the less you will have to ask later. This will result in a quicker and slicker consultation.

What would you ask next?

You should continue to gather information. Continue with open questions as these give the patient maximal opportunity to give you their history. Using closed questions too early on may ruin the patient's train of thought and you may miss something important.

You: "Can you tell me about any other symptoms?"

66 **Patient:** *"No, it's just the discharge and hearing loss."*

What would you ask next?

As the patient seems to have offered all that she is going to now would be a good time to explore her ideas, concerns and expectations (ICE). These should again be open questions to give the actor/patient the opportunity to divulge more information.

You: "Have you had any ideas about what's going on? Can you tell me about your main concerns? What thoughts had you had about how we might proceed from here?"

HISTORIES

66 **Patient:** *"I'm not sure what is causing this but I am worried that I'm going to lose my hearing permanently. I want something to make the ear discharge go away, it is starting to really get me down and I find it embarrassing."*

Tip - people may not wish to disclose their ideas and concerns for fear of looking silly. Often they have discussed it with family or searched the internet. If they are not too forth-coming with their worries a useful phrase to get them to open up is "a lot of people Google their symptoms and can see some worrying things. Have you seen anything that's worried you?"

What questions would you ask that might lead you to a diagnosis?

Now that you know the actor/patient's main ideas, concerns and expectations regarding the consultation and have given her ample opportunity to tell you about the history of her condition you can proceed onto focused, closed questions to help you make a diagnosis. Choose focused questions that either help you confirm the suspected diagnosis or rule out another diagnosis from the list of differentials. This is the point to ensure you specifically ask about the pertinent "red flags."

✏️ **Focussed Hearing Loss Questions**

You will want to know the exact onset of symptoms and the associated features that could alert you to any complications.
• Do you have any ear pain?
• Have you noticed any dizziness or vertigo?
• Has your hearing loss been progressive or does it fluctuate? Do you hear any added sounds or ringing in your ears?
• Have you had any facial weakness?
• Any fever or rigors?
• Any headaches, photophobia?
• Have you had any previous ear surgery?

---

66 **Patient:** *"I don't have any pain. I sometimes lose my balance and get a little bit disorientated. My hearing has been getting gradually worse, I don't get any ringing in my ears. I haven't experienced any of the other symptoms. I had a grommet as a child but I can't remember which side."*

What else would you like to ask?

Once you are happy that you fully understand the presenting complaint and the patient's concerns you should concisely run through the rest of the history to double check that you have not missed anything that could be relevant. You should cover PMH, DH, SH and a quick systems review. If everything has gone to plan then there should be no surprises here.

You: "Do you have any other medical conditions? Have you had any operations?"

66 **Patient:** *"No. I had glue ear when I was little and had a grommet inserted."*

You: "Do you have any allergies?"

❝ Patient: *"No."*

You: "Do you take any medications, either prescribed or bought over-the-counter?"

❝ Patient: *"I've just finished some ear drops from the GP, but they haven't helped. I don't take any regular medications."*

You: "Do you smoke/drink?"

❝ Patient: *"I don't smoke. I have a glass of wine every now and again."*

You: "What do you do for work? Who is there at home with you?"

❝ Patient: *"I'm a teaching assistant and I live my husband and 2 year old daughter."*

How would you close the scenario?

Now that you have come to the end of your history it is good practise to summarise back to the patient to ensure you have all the facts. This also allows her the opportunity to add/correct anything. After summarising you can check there is nothing else she wishes to add before thanking her and explaining what your management plan is.

You: "OK, just to check I haven't missed anything can I just clarify what you've told me". You have had persistent right sided ear discharge for the last year, it is offensive and occasionally bloody. You have also noticed some hearing loss and occasional dizziness. None of the medications from your GP have helped. You previously had glue ear and grommet insertion as a child. You are otherwise well and take no regular medications. Is this correct? Is there anything else you think I have missed?"

❝ Patient: *"No that all sounds right."*

Explain to the patient what would you like to do next?

You: "I would like to perform otoscopy to look for perforation and any white masses, classical of cholesteatoma. I would also examine the cranial nerves to exclude intracranial involvement. In order to assess signs of active infection, I will take an FBC, CRP and a swab for M,C&S. A CT scan will show extent of disease and can aid surgical planning."

SUMMARY

Your history should focus on the course of her symptoms and associated and negative features and highlight any symptoms indicating serious complications such as intracranial infection.

Cholesteatoma is a rare type of ear disease, most commonly affecting children or young adults. It can be congenital, or more commonly acquired secondary to recurrent ear infections. It is characterised clinically by recurrent ear infections and progressive hearing loss.

HISTORIES

Initial treatment is to treat any underlying infection with eardrops and regular aural suction. A CT will demonstrate extent of disease and help to plan the surgical approach. Surgery consists of a mastoidectomy. A closed mastoidectomy is performed via the ear canal or with a post-auricular incision for small cholesteatomas, radical mastoidectomy involves removing most of the mastoid for extensive disease and modified radical mastoidectomy preserves some of the middle ear bones and a synchronous tympanoplasty is performed.

😐 Actor Brief

You are Debbie Michaels, a 35-year-old woman. You have had a smelly discharge from your right ear for the last year, more recently your husband has commented that your hearing is getting worse. You are worried that the hearing loss is a sign of something serious. You have been referred to the ENT clinic by your GP after recurrent courses of antibiotics and eardrops have failed to improve your symptoms.

Presenting Complaint: You have had persistent offensive right ear discharge on and off for the last year. It is a thick yellow discharge with occasional bloody streaks. It smells very badly and you are struggling to deal with this. You have no ear pain. You have tried eardrops and antibiotics prescribed by the GP but the symptoms always return. Over the last month your husband has noticed you are increasing the volume on the television and struggling to hear phone conversations.

ICE: You are frightened by your hearing loss and are afraid it is permanent. The ear discharge is becoming embarrassing and has affected your self-confidence.

Significant PMH/DH/SH: You are a teaching assistant. You live with your husband and 2-year-old daughter. You have no allergies. You don't take any regular medication but have finished a course of antibiotic eardrops recently. As a child you had glue ear and grommet insertion. You are a non-smoker and have the occasional glass of wine.

TOP TIPS

➕ After initiating the presenting complaint, chronology of events and disease progression are important when dealing with long-term problems.

➕ When discussing the management plan be sure to address any immediate clinical issues such as chance of infection and then offer a longer-term solution.

➕ In this scenario it is important to demonstrate empathy regarding her hearing loss.

3.15 | Limping Child

Scenario

Your next patient in the orthopaedic clinic is Billy Hopkins. He has arrived with his mother. He is a 14-year-old boy who has been referred by the GP with a 3 week history of pain in the left knee and limping.
You have washed your hands and introduced yourself. Please take a history and suggest a management plan.

How would you begin?

Begin with an open question and allow the patient to explain as much as he feels able to. Let the patient speak freely and without interruption and listen actively to the history. You can ask the mother questions to clarify also.

You: "Can you tell me what has brought you into clinic?"

❝ Patient: *"I have a sore knee. It's been hurting for the last few weeks. I am supposed to play football every weekend but because of my knee I can't play anymore."*

What would you ask next?

You should continue to gather information. Continue with open questions at this stage as it is too soon to use closed questions and you may miss something important if you cut the patient off too early. Further open questions give the actor/patient another opportunity to disclose information.

You: "Tell me more about this pain?"

❝ Patient: *"It's in my left knee. It feels like a niggling pain all over my knee, it's a bit better when I'm sitting down. I can't remember how it started, it just happened. It is there all the time but it is getting worse. My mum said that I've been walking funny too."*

What would you ask next?

As the patient seems to have offered all that he is going to now would be a good time to explore his ideas, concerns and expectations (ICE). These should again be open questions to give the actor/patient the opportunity to divulge more information.

You: "What do you think is going on? What is your main concern? What were you expecting when you came here today?"

Tip: If the patient expressed an idea/concern/expectation earlier on, blindly asking about them in a rote fashion will make it seem as if you have not been listening. Instead reflect it back in your question.

You: "You said earlier that you like football and that you can't play, is that something that's been worrying you?"

Patient: *"Yes, I really want to know what is causing the pain so we can fix it and I can start playing football again."*

What questions would you ask that might lead you to a diagnosis?

Now that you know the actor/patient's main ideas, concerns and expectations regarding the consultation and have given him ample opportunity to tell you about the history of his condition you can proceed onto focused, closed questions to help you make a diagnosis.

Focussed Hearing Loss Questions

You will want to know the exact onset of symptoms and if there any associated features. In particular you want to know:
• Does the pain stay in the knee or does it move up and down the leg?
• Is the pain worse when you put weight on it?
• Do you have any pain in any other joints?
• Have you had a fever or any viral illnesses recently?
• Have you banged the knee or injured it in any way?
• Have you noticed any knee swelling?
• Does anything improve the pain or make it worse?
• Have you had anything like this before?
• Has anyone else in your family had a similar problem?

Patient: *"The pain stays in my knee, sometimes higher up in my leg hurts a bit too but not as much as my knee. It's worse when my weight is on it. I have no pain in any other joints and I haven't been unwell. I can't remember banging it and it has never been swollen. Nothing really makes it better aside from sitting down. This is the first time I've had anything like this. My mum said no one else has had any problems with their knee."*

What else would you like to ask?

Once you are happy that you fully understand the presenting complaint and the patient's concerns you should quickly run through the rest of the history to double check that you have not missed anything that could be relevant. In a child be sure to ask about school and the social situation.

You: "Do you have any other medical conditions? Have you had any operations?"

Patient: *"No."*

You: "Do you have any allergies?"

Patient: *"No."*

You: "Do you take any medications?"

Patient: *"No."*

You: "How is school going? What do you like to do in your spare time? Who lives at home

HISTORIES

with you?"

66 **Patient:** *"School is fine, I will take my GCSEs next year. I like playing computer games and I play football every weekend when my knee isn't hurting. I live my mum, dad and little sister."*

How would you close the scenario?

Now that you have come to the end of your history it is good practise to summarise back to the patient to ensure you have all the facts. This also allows him the opportunity to add/correct anything. After summarising you can check there is nothing else he wishes to add before thanking him and explaining what your management plan is.

You: "OK, just to check I haven't missed anything can I just clarify what you've told me. You have had left sided knee pain for the last 3 weeks. It occasionally travels up to the groin. It is worse on weight baring and has started to interfere with playing football. You mum has noticed you are limping. You have not been unwell and have suffered no trauma. Is this correct? Is there anything else you think I have missed?"

66 **Patient:** *"No that all sounds right."*

What is your differential diagnosis?

In a 14-year-old male my differential diagnosis includes:
• Slipped upper femoral epiphysis (SUFE)
• Transient synovitis
• Septic arthritis
• Perthe's disease

SUMMARY

Slipped upper femoral epiphysis (SUFE) is a condition that results in slippage of the epiphysis in relation to the femoral neck. It has a preponderance to affect the left hip and can be bilateral. It affects males more than females (3:2) and peaks in boys aged 13 years and girls 12 years. It is more common in those of African-Caribbean heritage and obese children. It can be associated with hypothyroidism, growth hormones disorders and previous radiotherapy to the hip.

Clinical presentation is often with isolated knee pain on the affected side but can present with hip pain or acutely with severe pain and inability to weight bear

In an acute SUFE patients should be made non-weight bearing to prevent worsening the severity of the slip and admitted to hospital for definitive treatment. The treatment of SUFE is always surgical. One option is percutaneous pinning to stabilise the epiphysis. Prophylactic surgical fixation of the contralateral leg is sometimes recommended. Post-operatively, physiotherapy and weight loss should be recommended.

HISTORIES

😐 Actor Brief

You are Billy Hopkins, a 14-year-old boy. Your mum, because of right-sided knee pain, has brought you to the orthopaedic clinic.

Presenting Complaint: For the last 3 weeks you have had a vague twinge in your right knee, it has got slightly worse. You have not been able to play football recently as it makes the pain worse. Prior to this you were fit and well and have never had any problems with your knee. You have not suffered any trauma. You don't have any other symptoms. Your mum has noticed that you are walking with a limp.

ICE: You are worried that you won't be able to play football any more. Your mother is concerned it is because she has pushed you to do more exercise because the school nurse has noticed you are overweight.

Significant PMH/DH/SH: You are at school and are doing well academically. You enjoy football, and you started playing for a local team every weekend to try and lose weight. You have no allergies and don't take any medication.

TOP TIPS

➕ It looks good in the exam if you can name a few classification systems- there is no need to learn them in great detail just the basics will suffice.

➕ There are a few clues in this history- left sided pain in an obese child with no history of trauma!

➕ When discussing radiological investigations, try to specify which views you want and what you are looking for.

HISTORIES

3.16 Loin Pain

Scenario

Your next patient is Michael Harris. He is a 42-year-old solicitor. He presented A&E with severe left sided abdominal/loin pain. He is in obvious distress. You have washed your hands and introduced yourself. Please take a history and suggest a management plan.

How would you begin?

Begin with an open question and allow the patient to explain as much as he feels able to. Allow the patient to speak uninterrupted and actively listen to the history.

You: "What has brought you into hospital?"

66 **Patient:** *"I have an agonizing pain in my left side. It's the worst pain I've ever felt."*

What would you ask next?

He's not given you much information so you should continue to gather information. It is too soon to focus your questions on this symptoms and you may miss other important information. Continue with open questions to give the actor/patient a further opportunity to disclose information.

You: "Can you tell me about any other symptoms?"

66 **Patient:** *"I've been sick a few times. But mainly it's just this pain."*

What would you ask next?

The patient's responses are short and concise as clearly he is in discomfort and therefore a concise historian. You don't want to unnecessarily prolong the consultation but you must ensure you don't cut any corners. This is where slick questioning comes into play. Explore his thoughts briefly before focusing your questions.

You: "What do you think is going on? What is your main concern? What were you expecting when you came here today?"

66 **Patient:** *"I don't know what it is, that's why I'm here! Can I please have something to get rid of this pain?"*

Tip: Clearly his initial expectation is to be pain-free, so asking his expectations at this point may aggravate him if it seems you are taking a history in a rote fashion. However, do not assume that he has no other expectations. Pain can cloud one's thought process, so you may need to re-visit some elements of the history once he is more comfortable.

What questions would you ask that might lead you to a diagnosis?

Now that you his presenting complaint you can proceed onto focused, closed questions to help you make a diagnosis.

> ✏️ **Focussed Loin Pain Questions**
> • A focused pain history will narrow down your differential list and guide you to other specific enquires about associated features.
> • Any pain when passing urine?
> • Have you noticed any blood in your urine or a change in colour?
> • Any change in how often you pass urine?
> • Have you felt feverish, cold or shaky?
> • Any lighted or dizziness?
> • Any problems opening your bowels?

❝ **Patient:** *"The pain starts in my back and moves down my left side into my groin. It came on out of the blue. It comes in waves of severe cramping pain. Sometimes, I think it has gone but then it keeps coming back again. I've never felt anything like this before. Nothing has touched the pain, the pain relief I have had hasn't made much difference. It is 10/10 severity. I have been passing urine fine all day, it looks normal. I haven't had any fevers or shakes. When the pain comes I feel a little light headed. My bowels are fine."*

What else would you like to ask?

Once you are happy that you fully understand the presenting complaint and the patient's concerns you should quickly run through the rest of the history to double check that you have not missed anything that could be relevant. You should cover PMH, DH, SH and a quick systems review.

You: "Do you have any other medical conditions? Have you had any operations?"

❝ **Patient:** *"I've got high blood pressure and I suffer from gout. My GP said I have borderline diabetes."*

You: "Do you have any allergies?"

❝ **Patient:** *"No."*

You: "Do you take any medications?"

❝ **Patient:** *"I take ramipril, simvastatin and allopurinol. But recently I haven't been taking them as I should."*

You: "Do you smoke/drink?"

❝ **Patient:** *"I smoke about 20 a day. I enjoy a few glasses of wine in the evenings."*

You: "What do you do for work? Who is there at home with you?"

❝ **Patient:** *"I'm a solicitor. I live on my own."*

How would you close the scenario?

Now that you have come to the end of your history it is good practise to summarise back to the patient to ensure you have all the facts. This also allows him the opportunity to add/correct anything. After summarising you can check there is nothing else she wishes to add before thanking her and explaining what your management plan is.

You: "OK, just to check I haven't missed anything can I just clarify what you've told me. You presented as an emergency with your first episode of sudden onset left sided abdominal pain that moves to your groin. The pain is intermittent and cramping in nature. You have vomited with the pain. You have had no problems passing urine. You have high blood pressure and gout, but don't always take your medication. You are not allergic to anything. Is this correct? Is there anything else you think I have missed?"

66 **Patient:** *"No."*

What is your differential diagnosis?

In a 42-year-old man my differential diagnosis includes:
• Left renal colic
• Leaking abdominal aortic aneurysm
• Urinary tract infection/ pyelonephritis
• Small bowel obstruction

Please explain your management plan to the patient

You: "My first priority is to try and make you more comfortable with some pain relief. I would like to do some blood tests and take a sample of your urine. I will also request an x-ray of your abdomen. Depending of the results of the tests, we may need to do a more detailed scan called a CT scan to look at your kidneys and urinary system. Have I explained that clearly or is there anything you'd like me to go over again?"

66 **Patient:** *"No, that all makes sense."*

SUMMARY

In a distressed patient the priority is obtain a clear history to enable you to request appropriate investigations and initiate treatment as quickly as possible.

Acute ureteric calculi is a common emergency presentation of abdominal pain. Renal calculi are more common in men than women and can be associated with a wide range of other conditions. A classical history is loin to groin pain in a restless patient with microscopic haematuria. Variations in presentation depend on the location and size of stone.

Small stones <5mm can often be managed conservatively with analgesia and fluids until the stone passes spontaneously. Larger stones can cause obstruction of the urinary tract with subsequent hydronephrosis and are likely to need intervention. Complications of renal calculi include obstruction of the urinary system leading to hydronephrosis, if this becomes infected it is called pyonephrosis. Recurrence rate of renal calculi is high, as high as 50% recurrence rate within 5 years of the first presentation.

HISTORIES

☺ **Actor Brief**

You are Michael Harris, a 42 year old solicitor. You presented to the emergency department with severe left sided abdominal pain. You live alone and smoke 20 cigarettes a day. You drink half a bottle of red wine most evenings.

Presenting Complaint: You developed sudden onset severe left sided abdominal pain, it is the worst pain you have experienced. It starts in your back and moves down the left side of your abdomen. Lying still makes it worse but you cannot get comfortable. It is intermittent in nature, coming in severe cramping waves. When the pain is at its worse it makes you vomit. You have never experienced this before. You have no problems passing urine or opening your bowels.

ICE: Your only concern is to get rid of the pain, you are rather preoccupied by this and frequently ask for pain relief during the consultation.

Significant PMH/DH/SH: You are a solicitor and live alone. You have no allergies. You have high blood pressure and occasional gout. Your GP has advised you to modify your lifestyle as you have borderline diabetes but you have not complied. You are on ramipril, simvastatin and allopurinol, however you often forget to take them. You have smoked 20 cigarettes a day for the last 15 years and drink half a bottle of wine most evenings.

TOP TIPS

✚ In a young patient presenting with their first episode of loin pain, it is important to exclude leaking AAA early as a differential diagnosis. Make sure you mention this in OSCE stations!

✚ When dealing with a patient in severe pain, it is important to reassure them and offer analgesia as early as possible.

✚ Medical comorbidities can alert you to the possible diagnosis. Gout can be associated with the less common uric acid stones.

3.17 | Right Iliac Fossa Pain

Scenario

Your next patient is Claire Dowson. She is an 18-year-old lady who has been referred by the out of hours GP with lower abdominal pain and vomiting. You have washed your hands and introduced yourself. Please take a history and suggest a management plan.

How would you begin?

Begin with an open question and allow the patient to explain as much as she feels able to. Try not to interrupt and actively listen to the history.

You: "Can you tell me what has brought you into hospital?"

66 **Patient:** *"I started with stomach pains yesterday and it's just getting worse. The pain started higher up in my stomach but now it has moved lower down and more to the right. I feel tired and sick."*

What would you ask next?

The patient has given you some good information here but avoid the temptation to use more focused questions too soon. You should continue to gather information. It is too soon to use close questions as you may miss something important. Use a further open question to give the actor/patient another opportunity to disclose information.

You: "Can you tell me about any other symptoms you have?"

66 **Patient:** *"I've been sick four times this evening and I don't feel well."*

What would you ask next?

As the patient seems to have offered all that she is going to now would be a good time to explore her ideas, concerns and expectations (ICE). These should again be open questions to give the actor/patient the opportunity to divulge more information.

You: "What do you think is going on? What is your main concern? What were you expecting when you came here today?"

66 **Patient:** *"The GP said it could be appendicitis. My brother had his appendix out a few years ago and he was in hospital for a week. I can't afford to take any time off university as I have exams coming up. I'm keen to go home as soon as possible."*

What questions would you ask that might lead you to a diagnosis?

Now that you know the actor/patient's main ideas, concerns and expectations regarding the consultation and have given her ample opportunity to tell you about the history of her condition you can proceed onto focused, closed questions to help you make a diagnosis.

HISTORIES

> 🖉 **Focussed Right Iliac Fossa Questions**
>
> • Any change in bowel habit? When the last time you opened your bowels?
> • Any urinary symptoms?
> • When was your last period?
> • Do you normally get pain in between your periods?
> • Have you noticed any vaginal discharge?
> • Does anything improve the pain or make it worse?
> • Have you had anything like this before?
> • How is your appetite? Do you feel hungry?
> • Have you eaten anything unusual? Is anyone else unwell?
> • When did you last have something to eat or drink?

❝ Patient: *"The pain is here all the time now, nothing makes it better. The GP gave me some pain relief but the pain has come back now. I opened my bowels yesterday and it was normal. I have no problem passing water. My last period was just over 2 weeks ago, I do normally get pain between periods but this is much worse and feels different. I've not eaten since this morning but I don't feel hungry. I had a Chinese takeaway on Saturday night but none of my housemates are unwell."*

What else would you like to ask?

Once you are happy that you fully understand the presenting complaint and the patient's concerns you should quickly run through the rest of the history to double check that you have not missed anything that could be relevant. You should cover PMH, DH, SH and a quick systems review.

You: "Do you have any other medical conditions? Have you had any operations?"

❝ Patient: *"No."*

You: "Do you have any allergies?"

❝ Patient: *"Penicillin gives me a rash."*

You: "Do you take any medications?"

❝ Patient: *"I am on the contraceptive pill."*

You: "Do you smoke/drink?"

❝ Patient: *"I don't smoke. But I probably drink too much alcohol on the weekends."*

You: "What do you do for work? Who is there at home with you?"

❝ Patient: *"I'm a student and I live with 3 other housemates in town."*

How would you close the scenario?

Now that you have come to the end of your history it is good practise to summarise back to the patient to ensure you have all the facts. This also allows her the opportunity to add/correct anything. After summarising you can check there is nothing else she wishes to add before thanking her and explaining what your management plan is.

You: "You came into hospital due to worsening abdominal pain, which started centrally and has moved down to the right. You have vomited four times and feel unwell. You haven't noticed any changes to your bowels or water works and your last period was 2 weeks ago. Is this correct? Is there anything else you think I have missed?"

66 **Patient:** *"No that all sounds right."*

What is your differential diagnosis?

In an 18-year-old female my differential diagnosis includes:
• Appendicitis
• Gastroenteritis
• Ovarian pathology- ruptured ovarian cyst
• Mittelschmerz
• Urinary tract infection

Please explain your management plan to the patient

It is important that you clearly explain your plan to the patient. Acknowledge that in a young woman there are many possible causes for abdominal pain which we need to investigate.

You: "In a young woman of your age there a few different possible causes for your pain. To narrow this down there are a few tests we need to do to help make a diagnosis. We need to take some blood tests and a urine sample. I would also like to get an ultrasound scan, this can look for an inflamed appendix and any other causes such as ovarian cysts. Until we have the test results back, I would like you not to eat or drink anything. We will give you pain relief and something to help with your sickness. Have I explained that clearly or is there anything you'd like me to go over again?"

66 **Patient:** *"I understand. Am I going to need an operation?"*

You: "It depends on the test results. From what you have told me there is a possibility this could be appendicitis. In which case we would need to do an operation to remove the appendix."

SUMMARY

This is a common presenting surgical complaint. When taking your history it is important to illicit any associated symptoms in order to narrow down your differential diagnosis. Thinking ahead it is useful to know when the patient last ate, as she may need to go to theatre depending on test results.

Acute appendicitis is one of the commonest causes of a surgical abdomen. The typical history is 12-24 hours of central abdominal pain, which radiates to the right iliac fossa.

Nausea and vomiting are common as is reduced appetite, while change in bowel habit is less common and should alert you to other diagnoses. It is also uncommon to have a high fever with appendicitis. The treatment is appendicectomy. Generally, this is performed laparoscopically unless there are contraindications such as multiple previous abdominal operations, the patient is very young and therefore access would be difficult, or if upon beginning laparoscopically it is impossible to safely remove the appendix.

☺ Actor Brief

You are Claire Dowson an 18-year-old student. You feel unwell and are worried about staying in hospital because you have exams coming up.

Presenting Complaint: You developed general central stomach pain yesterday which has progressively got worse. The pain is worse in your lower abdomen and worse on the right side. You have vomited 4 times and feel unwell. You saw the out of hours GP this evening who sent you into hospital. You don't have any other symptoms.

ICE: You are concerned that this may be appendicitis as your younger brother had this and required an operation. You are anxious about staying in hospital as you have exams coming up and don't want to take any time off university.

Significant PMH/DH/SH: You are a university student. You live with housemates have no other health problems. You are allergic to pencillin, it gives you a nasty rash. You don't smoke and binge drink on weekends.

TOP TIPS

➕ After using open questions you should focus the history in order to form a list of differential diagnoses

➕ Your management plan should include remaining nil by mouth as there is a possibility of taking her to theatre

➕ It is also important to explain you will give some pain relief and anti-emetics whilst waiting for investigations

HISTORIES

3.18 | Right Buttock Pain

Scenario

Your next patient is Martin Gray. He is a 58-year-old man who has been referred by the GP with right buttock pain, ongoing for the last 7 months and getting progressively worse. You have washed your hands and introduced yourself. Please take a history and suggest a management plan.

How would you begin?

Begin with an open question and allow the patient to explain as much as she feels able to. Try not to interrupt and actively listen to the history.

You: "Can you tell me what has brought you into clinic?"

66 **Patient:** *"My GP sent me because of this leg pain. I've had a pain in this right leg for a long time but recently it's been getting worse. It started to travel up to my right buttock too. I find myself unable to walk to the pub now because I have to keep stopping because of this pain."*

What would you ask next?

The patient has given a concise set of information but resist the temptation to focus on this just yet. Continue to gather using open questions, which gives the actor/patient another opportunity to disclose information.

You: "Can you tell me about any other symptoms?"

66 **Patient:** *"No I'm otherwise very well."*

What would you ask next?

You should always explore the patient's ideas, concerns and expectations (ICE). These should again be open questions to give the actor/patient the opportunity to divulge more information.

You: "What do you think is going on? What is your main concern? What were you expecting when you came here today?"

66 **Patient:** *"I don't know, my brother's got arthritis but he's a bit older than me. It's becoming quite a nuisance having to keep stopping when I go for a walk."*

What questions would you ask that might lead you to a diagnosis?

Now that you know the actor/patient's main ideas, concerns and expectations regarding the consultation and have given him ample opportunity to tell you about the history of his condition you can proceed onto focused, closed questions to help you make a diagnosis. These should include appropriate questioning of red flag symptoms.

You will want to know the exact onset of symptoms and what the symptoms actually are. In particular you want to know:

HISTORIES

✎ **Focussed Buttock Pain Questions**

• Where does the pain start? Where does it move to?
• How far can you walk before getting the pain? Has this distance changed recently?
• How long does it take the pain to go away after stopping activity?
• Can you describe the pain- is it burning or sharp etc?
• Does anything improve the pain or make it worse?
• Do you get any pain at rest?
• Do you have any colour change or skin changes on your leg?
• Do you have any change in sensation in your leg?
• Do you have any back pain? Have you noticed any change in your bowel or bladder function?
• How much is this interfering with your daily life?

❝ **Patient:** *"The pain starts in my right thigh at the back and moves up to my buttock, it doesn't really move anywhere else. I can walk halfway to the pub, which is about 300 yards, I used to have no problem walking there and back 2 months ago. It takes a good 15 minutes before I can continue. It is a cramping type pain, not really burning. The GP gave me some gabapentin but it made no difference and I tried a walking stick but it didn't help. It only hurts when I'm walking. I haven't noticed any skin changes. I have diabetes so I can't feel my toes very well anyway, which has got worse over the years. I haven't much pain in my back and my bowels and bladder are fine. It is becoming a real problem, I've started driving short distances and I don't go out as much as I used to. I have to get online delivery for my food shopping because I can't walk around the supermarket."*

What else would you like to ask?

Once you are happy that you fully understand the presenting complaint and the patient's concerns you should quickly run through the rest of the history to double check that you have not missed anything that could be relevant. You should cover PMH, DH, SH and a quick systems review.

You: "Do you have any other medical conditions? Have you had any operations?"

❝ **Patient:** *"I have sugar diabetes. I had a triple heart bypass 3 years ago, but my heart is fine now."*

You: "Do you have any allergies?"

❝ **Patient:** *"No."*

You: "Do you take any medications?"

❝ **Patient:** *"Yes. Aspirin, bisoprolol, metformin, simvastatin and ramipril."*

You: "Do you smoke/drink?"

66 **Patient:** *"I smoke about 30 roll ups a day. I enjoy a pint or two in the pub most evenings."*

You: "What do you do for work? Who is there at home with you?"

66 **Patient:** *"I own a newsagent. I live with my wife and my daughter lives just a few doors down."*

How would you close the scenario?

Now that you have come to the end of your history it is good practise to summarise back to the patient to ensure you have all the facts. This also allows him the opportunity to add/correct anything. After summarising you can check there is nothing else he wishes to add before thanking him and explaining what your management plan is.

You: "OK, just to check I haven't missed anything can I just clarify what you've told me. You have been experiencing cramping pain in your right buttock and thigh for the last 7 months. It is triggered by exercise, you have no pain at rest. The distance you can walk is around 300m but has decreased recently. The pain is relieved completely by rest. You have diabetes and had a heart bypass. You smoke 30 roll ups a day and drink a few pints most evenings. Is this correct? Is there anything else you think I have missed?"

66 **Patient:** *"No that all sounds right."*

What is your differential diagnosis?

In a 58-year-old male my differential diagnosis includes:
• Intermittent claudication
• Chronic venous insufficiency
• Deep venous thrombosis
• Sciatica
• Osteoarthritis

What advice would you give to the patient? How will you manage him initially?

You: "In the first instance we will need to get some tests to look at whether any of your blood vessels might be blocked and causing your symptoms. These will include an ultrasound of your legs and some blood tests to check your blood sugar. Our treatment will depend on what these show but certainly lifestyle modifications including quitting smoking, losing weight and reducing your alcohol intake are advisable. We will also need to improve your diabetes control and blood pressure. You already take a blood thinner which is good and if there is a significant blockage shown in one of the tests you might need an operation to either breakdown or bypass the blocked vessels, but we can discuss this further when we see you back following the tests."

66 **Patient:** *"Thank you that all makes sense."*

SUMMARY

The key to eliciting a vascular pain history is to enquire precisely about triggering factors, claudication distance and alleviation by rest.

Intermittent claudication most commonly affects the lower limb with the superficial femoral artery the most common site for atheromatous plaque formation. At least 50% of the vessel diameter must be reduced before symptoms develop. In the above scenario the thigh and buttock pain is caused by a stenosis in the aortoiliac vessels, when this is combined with erectile dysfunction it is known as Leriche's syndrome.

Interventional treatment options include percutaneous transluminal angioplasty and endovascular stenting particularly for recurrent or extensive stenosis. More radical surgical options such as iliofemoral and aortofemoral bypass have largely been replaced by the less invasive angioplasty.

😐 Actor Brief

You are Martin Gray, a 58-year old newsagent; you are married with one grown up daughter. You attend clinic alone after you saw your GP with worsening right leg pain.

Presenting Complaint: For the last 7 months you have had right leg pain. It starts in the back of your right thigh and radiates up to your right buttock. Walking brings it on. It has got worse in the last two months and you are able to walk increasingly shorter distances. Now you can only walk 300 yards before the pain stops you. Rest eases the pain. You have no other symptoms.

ICE: You are keen to have a solution to this pain as it is starting to interfere with your daily life. You cannot walk to the pub without stopping and cannot go food shopping in the supermarkets.

Significant PMH/DH/SH: You own a newsagent and live with your wife. You have type 2 diabetes and 3 years ago underwent a triple heart bypass. You have no allergies. You take aspirin, simvastatin, bisprolol, ramipril and metformin. You smoke 30 roll ups a day and have 3 or 4 pints of beer a day at your local pub.

TOP TIPS

➕ Risk modification is the first and crucial step in managing most types of vascular disease.

➕ Key features suggestive of a vascular type pain as opposed to musculoskeletal or neuropathic pain are pain worse on walking uphill, alleviated entirely by rest and specific claudication distance.

➕ When discussing a management plan, it is best to start with conservative measures then build up to surgical options in a structured fashion.

3.19 | Thigh Swelling

Scenario

Your next patient is William Smith. He is an 11-year-old boy who has been referred to your paediatric orthopaedics clinic with a four-week history of progressive right thigh swelling. Please take a history from William, and if appropriate, his mother Jennifer, and suggest a management plan. You have washed your hands and introduced yourself.

How would you begin?

Allow the patient to give an initial account uninterrupted, and show signs of active listening.

You: "William, can you tell me what's been going on?"

❝❝ **Patient:** *[Silence] William is timorous and doesn't want to open up to the doctor.*

You turn to Jennifer, his mother, who gives the following collateral history:

❝❝ **Mother:** *"Don't worry doctor, he's just being shy! About a month ago, William told me that he'd noticed some swelling in his right thigh after playing football. He's had knocks like that before and they've all got better on their own so I told him to not run around as much for the next few days. I was quite shocked when he told me last week that the swelling's got worse. I had a look and it's about twice as big as it was initially."*

What would you ask next?

You have established that the patient has a rapidly progressive swelling of the right thigh, and now need to elucidate any related symptoms. Although initially, and understandably, blasé about the presenting complaint, it's clear that the patient's mother is shocked and perhaps concerned at this change. It might be sensible to acknowledge this at this early stage to attain rapport.

You: "It sounds like this has all happened rather quickly, I imagine it's been quite strange for you both and so it's important that we get to the bottom of this. Has William mentioned any other problems?"

❝❝ **Mother:** *"Thanks doctor, it has all come around very quickly and with things being so busy at home I'm quite stressed at the moment anyway. He hasn't really said anything specific, but I think it's getting more painful for him, I've noticed he's started to limp over the last week or so. He also hasn't been going out to play with his school friends, which is quite unusual for him."*

What else would you like to ask?

Before asking closed questions to refine your differential diagnosis, it would be helpful to elucidate Jennifer's ideas, concerns and expectations.

HISTORIES

You: "Have you had any thoughts about what might be going on? Is there anything that you're worried about? What do you feel we can do to help you today?"

66   **Mother:** *"Well, to begin with I thought it was probably just a football injury that would go away quite quickly. It's a bit strange that it hasn't but I still think the GP over-reacted by sending us all the way up here! I suppose my only real concern is that William is due to start at the high school on Monday and if he's limping around I don't want him to be a target for bullies. William's not really worried about anything, he just wants to get back to playing football with his friends! The timing's so difficult that I just want to get things sorted. Surely you can just prescribe us some painkillers and things will get better in the next few weeks?"*

What can you ask to reach a diagnosis?

By taking a comprehensive collateral history, you now have a good idea of the nature of the presenting complaint and its effects on William's personal and family life, and have established rapport with his mother. You should now use closed and focused questions to refine your differential diagnosis.

Pain history using SOCRATES: focus on the timing of the pain and exacerbating and relieving factors.
Presence of systemic symptoms e.g. weight loss, night sweats, fevers.

66   **Mother:** *"After he started limping I spoke to the GP and he recommended some paracetamol and seeing if it all settled. We gave that a go but it doesn't seem to have helped William. My ex-husband suggested giving him some ibuprofen but I know it can do funny things to your stomach so we haven't tried that yet. The only thing that seems to make it worse is walking and running and he's been doing less and less of that recently. William's always limping now so I imagine the pain's pretty constant. He's been fine otherwise. He does get up in the night, he's mentioned that the pain sometimes wakes him up, but hasn't had any sweats or fevers at all."*

What else would you like to ask?

You should now have a clearer picture of the exact nature of the presenting complaint and its functional implications. Complete your history by covering William's past medical, drug and social history and using systems review.

You: "Does William have any other health problems?"

66   **Mother:** *"He's had asthma for years but he uses his inhalers and it seems quite well controlled. Otherwise he's absolutely fine."*

You: "Are there any health problems that run in the family?"

66   **Mother:** *"Not that I can think of."*

You: "Is William taking any medications prescribed by a doctor?"

HISTORIES

❝ Mother: *"Only salbutamol and montelukast inhalers for his asthma."*

How would you close the scenario?

If you feel you have obtained all pertinent verbal information from William and his mother, synthesise the history you've taken so far and repeat this back to the pair. A clear summary will allow you to pick up on any ambiguous points and demonstrate your attentive listening to build rapport.

You: "William first noticed a swelling in his right thigh four weeks ago after playing football. This swelling has roughly doubled in size over the last month, and in the last week, Mum has noticed that William has been limping and hasn't been as willing as usual to go out and see his school friends. Mum's concerned about the fact this hasn't gone away despite rest and painkillers, and about the implications any injury might have on his transition to secondary school. William has a long-standing history of asthma but this is well controlled with salbutamol and montelukast inhalers. Have I missed anything out?"

❝ Mother: *"No doctor, that's exactly right."*

What is your differential diagnosis?

In an 11 year-old boy with new onset progressive thigh swelling and a recent limp, you must retain a high index of suspicion for osteosarcoma.
Other disorders to exclude are:
• Ewing sarcoma.
• Paediatric osteomyelitis.
• Benign tissue growths e.g. lipoma

Please explain your management plan to the patient and his mother.

Given William's shyness and a potentially traumatic diagnosis ahead, this presents a real challenge. Be clear in explaining the nature of and rationale behind your proposed investigations.

You: 'There are several problems that might explain both the progressive thigh swelling and William's recent problems with walking and running. At this stage, I'd like to perform some blood tests and obtain some X-rays of William's right leg and chest. These will give us some valuable information and help us to get to the bottom of what's been causing these problems. We'll need to perform these tests today so I'm afraid that you'll have to stay at the hospital a little while longer. We'll meet up again later to discuss the test results.'

❝ Mother: *'That's all well and good doctor, but I've got to get home to look after the kids! Surely we could do these tests another day?"*

It's clear that William's mother has yet to grasp the gravity of the situation and this gives you an opportunity both to demonstrate the urgency of the problem and break bad news in a sensitive and empathic manner.

Discuss the possibility of an osteosarcoma diagnosis with William and his mother.

You: "I'm sorry Mrs. Smith, and appreciate that this must be very frustrating for you. We'll do everything we can to speed things up, but from our point of view, our priority is working

HISTORIES

out exactly what is causing this swelling.

Tip: It will be difficult for the mother to hear the word 'cancer' so you should avoid it coming out of the blue. Appropriate body language and a serious but empathetic tone of voice will help signal that what you are dealing with is not trivial.

You: "There are many possible causes but we have to make sure that we don't miss anything important." Given William's age, one of the things that I'd like to rule out is something sinister. Do you know what I mean by when I say 'something sinister'?"
Tip - If possible, get her to say the word by guiding her to it. The word 'cancer' does need to be said, and you should not use any euphemisms.

66 **Mother:** *"Oh my god, do you mean this is cancer?!"*

You: "We are not sure yet, but one of the things this could be is a type of cancer affecting the thigh bone. This is clearly not something anyone wants to hear, may I go on?

Tip: By asking her permission to continue you show empathy for the bad news and also check she is ready to hear what you have to say next.

66 **Mother:** *"Er this is such a shock but yes, go on."*

You: "Performing the tests today will quickly provide us with an answer and help us to work out how best to treat William. I know this is a lot to take in and that you may not have been expecting that and you may have many questions either now or later. I will be happy to answer them at any time. Is there anything you'd like me to go over again now?"

66 **Mother:** *"It is a real shock, I can't think of anything right now but I want to get the tests as soon as possible."*

SUMMARY

This scenario is complicated by your reliance on a collateral history, a challenging three-way dynamic and a serious diagnosis. It is important to continue to engage both William and his mother throughout the consultation. At the point of explaining the possibility of a cancer diagnosis you should consider whether it is appropriate to have this conversation in front of William. It may be better to have that conversation without the child in the room, and allow his mother to discuss it with him at a later point. It is better to check with the parent at the appropriate point whether she wishes to have William present. If accompanied by an appropriately serious tone of voice, she should hopefully pick up on what you are implying and ask him to wait outside.

Be proactive in addressing Mrs. Smith's concerns about the rapid progression of the swelling, William's upcoming transition to secondary school, and her desire to return home to look after her other children, while emphasising the need to perform tests soon to rule out a worrying diagnosis.

☺ Actor Brief

You are Jennifer Smith, mother of William, a shy 11 year-old boy who is due to start at secondary school in four days time. William first mentioned some swelling in his right thigh a month ago after playing football and you are anxious to address the problem quickly so that you can return home to look after your three other children, currently under the care of your ex-husband.

Presenting Complaint: Four-week history of progressive right thigh swelling. William first noticed the swollen area after playing football and you told him it would probably settle down in a few days and that he didn't need to worry. However, more recently, when you were talking to him about an upcoming football match, William mentioned that the swelling had got worse. You went to see the GP last week, who made a referral to the orthopaedics clinic and suggested William try some paracetamol in the meantime. In the past week, you've noticed that William has started to limp and, unusually for him, hasn't wanted to play out with his school friends.

ICE: You think the GP who made the referral has probably over-reacted as this seems likely to be a football-related injury that will simply get better in time. However, the emergence of this new limp is a source of concern as William is due to start at secondary school in two weeks and you're worried it could lead to some bullying.

Significant PMH/DH/FH/SH: William was diagnosed with asthma aged 6 but this is well controlled with salbutamol and montelukast inhalers. He has no known drug allergies and is the third of your four children. As a busy working Mum, you want to resolve this issue as soon as possible to ensure a prompt return home.

TOP TIPS

➕ Osteosarcomas can often be missed by GPs who mistake the swelling in an otherwise well individual for a muscular injury or possibly a DVT in older patients. It should be considered in any patient with progressive swelling around a long-bone.

➕ Explaining things in a step-wise manner is key and using sign-posting and warning shots will help you to prepare the patient and his mother for the unexpected news.

HISTORIES

3.20   Knee Pain

Scenario

Mr. Jones is a 73-year-old man who you are seeing in clinic after being referred by the GP with worsening left knee pain, which has begun to prevent him from carrying out activities of daily living. You have washed your hands and introduced yourself. Please take a history and suggest a management plan.

How would you begin?

Introduce yourself and check you have the right patient.

You: "Hello, I'm Dr. X and I'm the surgical SHO. May I just check, are you Mr. Jones?"

Begin with an open question and allow the patient to explain as much as he feels able to. A friendly facial expression, tone of voice, and body language are all much more important than the semantics of the words you use. Allow the patient to speak uninterrupted and use active listening whilst they give you the history.

You: "I understand your GP has referred you to me; can you tell me what's been going on?"

> 66   **Patient:** *"It's my knee. My left one. It's been giving me a fair bit of grief for years since the accident but recently it's gotten so bad I can barely get about the house."*

What will you ask next?

You are acknowledging that you are interested in the whole story but probing more about the current presenting complaint.

You: "I'd like to hear more about the accident but can you first tell me more about your recent problems walking."

> 66   **Patient:** *"Well I do all the shopping for me and the missus but over the past year my left knee has been getting worse and worse. And now, over the past few months at the end of the day I can barely make it up the stairs to bed. It keeps me up at night at times. I've always been pretty independent but the painkillers my GP has given me aren't working much."*

What will you ask next?

Take the opportunity to demonstrate empathy and also explore the patient's concerns.

You: "It sounds like things have been difficult for you, is there anything you're particularly worried about?"

> 66   **Patient:** *"My wife and I don't want to go into a care home. We manage fine but this knee is making it hard for me to get the shopping in and we have no relatives*

nearby. I'm worried about what would happen to us and I don't want to lose my independence."

What will you ask next?

Now is a good time to focus on specific questions while thinking about what your differential diagnosis might be.

🖉 Focussed Knee Pain Questions

• What was the accident you had?
• Any more recent injuries to the knee?
• Any previous operations on the knee?
• When is the pain worse?
• What makes the pain better?
• Does the knee swell up?
• Does the knee give way?
• Any unintentional weight loss recently? In this age group it is worth ruling out any primary or secondary malignancy that could be affecting the bone.
• Any recent fever/hot-cold flashes? Although this is unlikely to be an acute condition, always rule out infective causes such as septic arthritis.

---

66 **Patient:** *"I fell off my motorbike 20 years ago and although I got patched up it's never been the same since. The pain is worst after I've been up and about all day on my feet. Resting eases it and moving about worsens it, the painkillers help a bit but less so now. It swells up a good few times a week, more often when I've done a bit too much. Its given way a few times when I've been hurrying down the stairs. I've been otherwise well and haven't had any weight loss or fevers."*

What else would you ask about?

Having established a good history of the knee pain it is now appropriate to screen through the remaining history.

You: "Do you have any other medical problems, allergies or take any tablets for anything?"

66 **Patient:** *"I have high blood pressure but I'm on tablets and the GP says it is fine, I don't have any allergies."*

You: "I'd like to ask about your general circumstances. You said you live with your wife in a house with stairs at the moment. Do you smoke or drink alcohol?"

66 **Patient:** *"I've never smoked. I have a couple of pints on Saturdays down the rugby club."*

How would you close the consultation?

You: "Mr. Jones, please correct me if I have misunderstood anything but as I understand it, you've had left knee pain for 20 years since a motorbike accident but which has progressively been worse in the last year, especially the last few months. This has been waking you up at night and is often worse at the end of the day and it is now interfering in your day to day activities. It swells up most days and has given way on you on several occasions. You suffer with high blood pressure but this is under control. You've been managing well at home until more recently and are worried the knee will affect your independence."

What is your diagnosis and what are your main differentials?

You: "In this patient my main differential is osteoarthritis of the left knee. Important differentials to rule out would be malignancy, infection (septic arthritis) and although unlikely given the history, any fracture."

Please explain your management options to the patient

You: "Mr. Jones, it seems very likely that you have arthritis in the left knee joint. How much do you know about arthritis?

❝❝ Patient: *"That's just the aches and pains of getting old isn't it?"*

You: "In a way you could explain it like that but it is really more the wear and tear of the cartilage lining of the knee. This cartilage allows the knee to glide smoothly as it moves. As the cartilage wears out, and this can be worsened by old injuries such as yours, the bone grinds directly on the other bone causing pain. This explains why you experience more pain as you go through the day. Tell me, what pain-killers have you tried so far?

❝❝ Patient: *"Co-codamol, but they only take the edge off."*

You: "What were you hoping to find out in this appointment with me today?"

❝❝ Patient: *"Can you give me a joint injection to make the pain go away?"*

You: "We can consider a joint injection but will need to get some up to date x-rays first and please understand an injection won't cure the arthritis."

❝❝ Patient: *"So what do I do now doc?"*

You: "Well when we treat arthritis such as yours we try non-surgical options first, such as painkillers, physiotherapy and joint injections. But these treatments just help control the symptoms. Ultimately once the arthritis is so severe that it prevents you from leading your life in the way you want to we consider the surgical option: a knee replacement. It sounds like you've tried painkillers already and they don't seem to be helping much. We may need to discuss the idea of surgery to replace the knee joint. Do you have any questions at this stage?"

❝❝ Patient: *"If I have this operation, when can I start walking?"*

You: "The same day if all goes as planned however you may need crutches or a frame for a few days until you feel steady on your feet with the physios."

❝❝ Patient: *"OK, well lets get the x-rays and then I'll need to have a think about an operation."*

You: "Absolutely."

SUMMARY

Your summary should include important positives and negatives that allow you to identify this is osteoarthritis and not other conditions. There should be clear indications of when the pain affects the patient and how this is eased/worsened. A timeline should be established. Important in all orthopaedic histories is the effect the patient's symptoms are having on their day to day life, independence, hobbies and responsibilities.

OA is common in older age groups and commonly affects the hips, knees and hands although most joints in the body can be affected. A history of trauma to a joint can accelerate the onset of OA.

😐 Actor Brief

You are Mr. Glyn Jones, 73 years old and suffering with severe arthritis of the left knee. You are generally in good health but are not keen on hospitals and are worried you will lose your ability to care for yourself and your wife.

General Information: You are anxious and simplistically hoping for an easy quick solution to the knee pain. It takes methodical explanation to help you understand a knee replacement is indicated.

Presenting Complaint: 1 year worsening left knee pain on a background of chronic knee troubles following a motorbike accident 20 years ago. Worse on movement and towards the end of the day. Stairs are especially troublesome. Occasionally the pain keeps you up at night. No weight loss or fevers.

ICE: Worried about loss of independence and being put in a care home. Hoping there is some quick solution to the knee pain that will allow you to get home quickly. Later on when management discussion occurs - hoping a joint injection will 'fix' the knee.

Significant PMH/DH/SH: Hypertension under control. NKDA. Non smoker, couple pints/wk. Lives with wife in house with stairs. No walking aids.

Special Instructions: If the subject of a knee replacement (surgery) is broached abruptly rather than being guided to it via non-surgical options first, become flustered and angry demanding medication to 'fix the knee so you can go home to your wife'.

TOP TIPS

➕ Ensure your questions allow you to differentiate between OA, RA, Gout and septic arthritis and trauma.

➕ Orthopaedic conditions often have a huge impact on activities of daily living/independence – make sure this is covered in either ICE or social history questions.

HISTORIES

HISTORIES

Made in the USA
Charleston, SC
01 August 2016